Patient Compliance: Sweetening the Pill

Patient Compliance: Sweetening the Pill

Edited by

Dr Madhu Davies and Dr Faiz Kermani

'Patient compliance is a multidimensional, multinational, and multidisease state problem.'
Dr Jane Chin

GOWER

Published by
Gower Publishing Limited
Gower House
Croft Road
Aldershot
Hampshire GU12 3HR
England

Gower Publishing Company
Suite 420
101 Cherry Street
Burlington,
VT 05401-4405
USA

British Library Cataloguing in Publication Data
Patient compliance : sweetening the pill
1. Patient compliance
I. Davies, Madhu II. Kermani, Faiz
615.5

ISBN-10: 0 566 08658 1
ISBN-13: 978-0-566-08658-8

Library of Congress Control Number: 2006935176

Typeset in Bembo by IML Typographers, Birkenhead, Merseyside
Printed in Great Britain by TJ International Ltd, Padstow, Cornwall

Contents

List of Figures and Tables

FIGURES

TABLES

List of Abbreviations

ACE	angiotensin-converting enzyme
ACEI	angiotensin-converting enzyme inhibitor
ADME	absorption, distribution, metabolism and excretion
API	active pharmaceutical ingredient
ARB	angiotensin II antagonist
AIHW	Australian Institute of Health and Welfare
AusDiab Study	Australian Diabetes, Obesity and Lifestyle Study
BSE	bovine spongiform encephalopathy
CDSMC	Chronic Disease Self-Management Course
CI	confidence intervals
CMO	Chief Medical Officer
CNAM	Caisse Nationale d'Assurance Maladie
COPD	chronic obstructive pulmonary disease
CRA	clinical research associate
CRO	clinical research organization
CV	curriculum vitae
CVD	cardiovascular disease
DARTS	Diabetes Audit and Research in Tayside, Scotland
DOT	directly observed therapy
DTC	direct-to-consumer
EPR	enhanced permeation and retention
EPP	Expert Patients Programme
EXCEL	Expanded Clinical Evaluation of Lovastatin
4S	Simvastatin Survival Trial
FDA	Food and Drug Administration
GCP	good clinical practice
GDP	gross domestic product
GP	general practitioner
HAM-D	Hamilton Rating Scale for Depression
HIV	human immunodeficiency virus
HPMC	hydroxypropylmethylcellulose
HRT	hormone replacement therapy
INN	international non-proprietary name
IOF	International Osteoporosis Foundation
IIT	investigator-initiated trial
IT	information technology

ITT	intention-to-treat
IVR	Interactive Voice Response
KOL	key opinion-leader
LEEF	Les enterprises du médicament
LDL	low-density lipoprotein
LHRH	luteinizing hormone-releasing hormone
LMCA	Long-Term Medical Conditions Alliance
LOI	letter of intent
MeMo	Medicines Monitoring Unit
MEMS	medication event monitoring system
MMR	measles, mumps and rubella
MI	myocardial infarction
MSL	medical science liaison
NDA	New Drug Application
OCP	oral contraceptive pill
OECD	Organization for Economic Cooperation and Development
OTC	over-the-counter
PA	physician's assistant
PCT	primary care trust
PDA	Personal Digital Assistant
PGLA	polylactic acid-polyglycolic acid copolymer
PRISM (study)	Platelet Receptor Inhibition in Ischaemic Syndrome Management (study)
PP	polypropylene
PTP	press-through pack
PVA	polyvinyl acetate
PVC	polyvinyl chloride
PVDC	polyvinylidine chloride
QALY	quality-adjusted life-year
QoL	quality of life
R&D	research and development
RCT	randomized controlled trial
RES	reticuloendothelial system
SHA	strategic health authority
SMS	short message service
SSRI	selective serotonin reuptake inhibitor
TB	tuberculosis
WHO	World Health Organization
WOSCOPS	West of Scotland Coronary Prevention Study

List of Contributors

Alan Blaskett is the International SOS Group Marketing Director of Pharma Services and drew on his experiences to write his contribution to this book. Over the past decade, Alan has worked within the pharmaceutical industry, specializing in the delivery of patient support and compliance initiatives. Initially working with Roche, he developed hands-on experience developing and implementing a programme to support patients prescribed the weight-loss medication, Xenical. In his work with International SOS approximately 25 programmes have been initiated across a variety of markets and therapeutic areas.

Mike Bradburn is a Consultant Biostatistician at PAREXEL International, UK. He is involved in a wide range of trials including oncology, virology and dermatology, and has experience in all statistical aspects of clinical research. Prior to joining PAREXEL, Mike was a statistician at Cancer Research UK in Oxford, during which time he co-authored two book chapters and more than 20 articles in medical journals. Mike has ten years' experience of working as an applied statistician and holds a degree in Statistics as well as a Masters degree in Statistics with Applications in Medicine.

Dr Bill Byrom, BSc, PhD is a Product Strategy Director at ClinPhone, UK, with responsibilities for new areas of technology application within clinical trials and healthcare. Bill joined the pharmaceutical industry in 1991 after completing a PhD in disease control simulation at Strathclyde University, and has worked in a number of roles within Statistics, Clinical Development and International Marketing. Bill is the author of over 40 published articles in professional journals and publications.

Dr Jane Chin is President of the Medical Science Liaison Institute, USA and helps biopharmaceutical companies transform field-based medical science teams into competitive assets. She is widely published in field-based medical programme topics, including training, compliance, competitive intelligence and performance metrics. Jane has over a decade of pharmaceutical industry experience spanning analytical R&D, sales and medical affairs. She gained her BS in Microbiology from Cornell University and her PhD in Biochemistry from Roswell Park Cancer Institute/University of Buffalo. Jane is also a certified Competitive Intelligence Professional.

Dr Madhu Davies is a Consultant in Pharmaceutical Medicine. She joined the pharmaceutical industry in 1993 after several years in clinical practice and has retained her interest in what makes the patient 'tick', which critically includes the complex area of compliance and the issues around it.

Dr Brian Edwards is a Senior Medical Adviser and deputy qualified person in pharmacovigilance at Johnson & Johnson Pharmaceutical Research and Development. Formerly he was a Senior Director in PAREXEL International's Medical Services responsible for medical input into clinical trials and post-marketing pharmacovigilance, including consultancy on risk–benefit and crisis management, advice about pharmacovigilance processes and strategy, and overseeing the implementation of pharmacovigilance contracts for various clients. Before joining PAREXEL, Dr Edwards was a Senior Medical Assessor in the UK Pharmacovigilance Assessment Group of the Medicines Control Agency (MCA) and was responsible for the assessment of major drug/vaccine safety issues. He also served on the panel, appointed by the UK Faculty in Pharmaceutical Medicine, overseeing the 'Drug Safety Surveillance' module as part of higher medical training for pharmaceutical medicine in the UK.

Tanwen Evans works for PAREXEL, a global contract research organization that offers a range of services to assist the pharmaceutical, biotech and medical device industries in bringing new products to market. Currently, she is Senior Project Manager in the Recruitment Services Group, developing sophisticated, ethical-approved programmes that enhance patient recruitment and retention in clinical trials and motivate and engage the investigators involved. Her career to date has given her a thorough appreciation of how optimal compliance is key to so many facets of the pharmaceutical industry, from a patient's compliance to medication to a physician's compliance to a study protocol.

Dr Dyffrig Hughes BPharm MSc PhD MRPharmS is a Senior Research Fellow in pharmacoeconomics at the Centre of Economics and Policy in Health at the University of Wales, UK. Dyffrig's research interests are in quantifying the pharmacological, clinical and health economic impact of patient non-compliance.

Dr Shane Jackson PhD is a National Institute of Clinical Studies Research Fellow at the Unit for Medication Outcomes Research and Education (UMORE), University of Tasmania, Australia. Shane is a practising community pharmacist and is active in the area of medication management reviews. His research interests lie in promoting the uptake of evidence in practice and promoting the safe and efficacious use of anticoagulants.

Dr Richard Kay is an independent statistical consultant and trainer. He gained his PhD from the London School of Hygiene and Tropical Medicine in 1976, working under the supervision of Peter Armitage. He then spent 13 years in academia at the universities of Salford, Heidelberg and Sheffield, undertaking teaching and research. In 1989 he left his position at Sheffield University to establish S-Cubed, a small company offering consultancy, training and data analysis services to the pharmaceutical industry. Following a period of growth he merged S-Cubed with PAREXEL International in 1997. Until recently, Richard was Vice President at PAREXEL heading up the worldwide Biostatistics and Programming group. He now works as an independent statistical consultant and trainer.

Caroline Kelham, Geraldine Mynors and Joanne Shaw work at Medicines Partnership. This is an initiative, funded by the English Department of Health, aimed at enabling patients to get the most out of medicines by involving them as partners in decisions about treatment, to the extent that they want it, and supporting them in medicine-taking. The team have been working with stakeholders including health professionals, patients, academics, government and the pharmaceutical industry to identify successful strategies and integrate a partnership model throughout the healthcare sector in England.

Dr Faiz Kermani PhD was formerly European Marketing Manager, Chiltern International, but now works for a medical communication agency in London. Faiz has previously worked in business development at CMR International, examining R&D productivity issues for pharmaceutical industry clients. He has also worked as a research analyst for a Danish healthcare consultancy, Informedica A/S, focusing on global pharmaceutical pricing and parallel importation. He holds a PhD in Immunopharmacology from St Thomas's Hospital, London and a first-class honours degree in Pharmacology with Toxicology from King's College, London.

Dr Akira Kusai PhD is the Director of Pharmaceutical Development Laboratories, Sankyo Company Ltd., Japan where he has worked since he gained his MS from the Faculty of Science, Osaka University in 1973. He was awarded a PhD from the Faculty of Pharmaceutical Science, Kyoto University in 1987. Between 1980 and 1982 he spent time with Dr W.I. Higuchi at the College of Pharmacy, University of Michigan as a visiting research associate. He has authored and co-authored more than 80 articles, abstracts and presentations. Current scientific and research interests include the design and development of solid and parenteral dosage forms and novel drug delivery systems.

Professor Thomas M. MacDonald is Professor of Clinical Pharmacology and Pharmacoepidemiology at the division of Medicine and Therapeutics and Community Health Sciences, University of Dundee and Honorary Consultant Physician at Ninewells Hospital and Medical School. Tom's major interests and expertise are cardiovascular disease and pharmacoepidemiology. He is actively involved in a number of major research projects and has published over 230 papers on cardiovascular and pharmacoepidemiological topics.

Janice MacLennan is the Principal Director of both St Clair Solutions and St Clair Consulting. She is an internationally recognized thought leader in strategic brand planning. St Clair Solutions is the organization behind the design, development and introduction of SCRxIBE – a leading strategic brand planning tool. St Clair Consulting is a strategic marketing consultancy. Janice has directed marketing consultancy assignments for multinational healthcare companies, working with them in the USA and internationally. These assignments have included developing, testing and supporting strategic brand planning processes from which the material for her latest book, Brand Planning for the Pharmaceutical Industry (2004), has been derived.

Catherine Narayan-Dubois is a pharmacist. After obtaining her degree from the University of Limoges, France, Catherine moved into the pharmaceutical industry where she gained experience in the field of international regulatory affairs.

Brendan O'Rourke is a Senior Trainer for the Expert Patient Programme, UK. His background is in community development, project management and human rights work and he has worked for several charities. Brendan joined the UK National Health Service in 2002 as one of the first self-management Senior Trainers for the Expert Patients Programme, developing partnerships and organizing self-management courses for people with long-term conditions in south-east London and Kent. Now a Trainer of Lead Trainers for EPP, he (with colleagues) has a national remit to oversee the training and quality framework for self-management. This has been developed to ensure consistent practices and quality standards across the NHS and in the voluntary sector. Consistent standards are designed to ensure a continuation of quality in course delivery when EPP is mainstreamed throughout the NHS by 2008.

Dr John Parkinson was formerly Client Services Director at the Medicines Monitoring Unit, Dundee, UK, and is now at the MHRA. John gained his PhD in Biochemistry from the University of Liverpool and has worked both within the pharmaceutical industry and as a consultant to it in areas that include advertising, PR and medical education. In 1995 he joined the pharmacoepidemiology/database group, MEMO, at the University of Dundee, as Client Services Director where he was responsible for managing the relationship with study sponsors and users of data. He has lectured widely on many aspects of pharmacoepidemiology, including patient compliance, or lack of it, as well as record-linkage and confidentiality/privacy enhancing technologies issues. He joined the (UK) Medicines and Healthcare products Regulatory Authority (MHRA) in September 2005 as Group Manager for GPRD, the world's largest longitudinal primary care database.

Professor Gregory Peterson holds a personal Chair in Pharmacy at the University of Tasmania, Australia. He has a background in community, hospital and academic pharmacy. His research interests centre on improving the use of medicines, and he has led many community and hospital projects directed at improving the use of medications and patient outcomes. He also has research interests in the use of information and communications technology to improve the safety and efficacy of healthcare delivery, including the use of medications.

David B. Stein BSc is Product Strategy Director, ClinPhone, UK. David has worked in pharmaceutical technologies for over 20 years in a variety of roles. He has established the data management department for a medium-sized CRO, founded a start-up company providing mobile patient-reported outcomes and has created software for pharmaceutical post-marketing applications used in several countries. At ClinPhone, David is a Product Strategy Director with responsibilities for new areas of technology application within clinical trials and healthcare.

Dr Li Wei PhD holds a Special Training Fellowship in the Health Service and Health of the Public Research Award from MRC, UK and works with the Medicines Monitoring Unit, Dundee, UK. After graduating in Medicine from the Anhui Medical University, China, Li obtained an MSc in Epidemiology from the University of Aberdeen and a PhD in Pharmacoepidemiology from the University of Dundee. She joined the Medicines Monitoring Unit in August 2000 as a statistician/epidemiologist.

Dr Graham Wylie is Managing Director of the Clinical Trials Division of Healthcare at Home – a major private provider of home care services in the UK. Having qualified in

Pharmacology and Medicine, he joined Pfizer in 1989 where he worked in a variety of roles. He started by managing clinical trials in Europe, then moved to New York to run enterprise-wide business re-engineering programmes relating to trials data and finally returned to Europe to provide general management services to the clinical development organization. In 1999 he joined PAREXEL – a global contract research organization – as Medical Director for Northern Europe, before becoming their Vice President of Account Management for the company's Clinical Research Services in Europe. In 2005 he joined the board of Healthcare at Home with the specific remit of accelerating their embryonic clinical trials business as well as utilizing his broad experience across the business generally.

Preface

Despite the advances in producing new medicines, healthcare improvements depend to a large extent on patient compliance. In recent years, growing efforts have been made by all parties in the healthcare sector to find optimal therapeutic approaches for patients. A range of technologies and product strategies has been developed to address the problems concerning patient compliance, but these are not the only approaches needed. Equally important is a thorough understanding of patients themselves and their attitudes to the medicines they take. Social, economic and cultural issues all play a part in determining patient compliance. Furthermore, such factors can vary widely amongst populations across the world and so care must be taken in making assumptions on how a particular medicine will be accepted in different countries.

In order to demonstrate the growing importance of this field, this book brings together a broad range of views from authors with interests in all aspects of compliance. The authors provide their own working definitions of compliance and then go on to discuss this in the context of their field of interest. There is inevitably some overlap but this is both necessary and unavoidable in a book of this type. However, we hope that, by providing a range of views from different experts in the field, the discussion on patient compliance can be widened so as to encourage further interest in the subject.

The book has been divided into four Parts, which seek to define what compliance is and why it is important to patients, health professionals and the pharmaceutical industry. To stimulate the discussion of this subject, two examples of the challenges of compliance from very different disease areas and countries are provided. In addition there are discussions on how compliance might be built in from the outset of therapy and, finally, a vision of the future in which the patient leads the way on these themes. Hopefully this will provide an easy reference on the subject for a variety of readers interested in compliance issues – ranging from those who seek to 'dip into' it for information on a specific aspect of compliance to those who seek to read it from start to finish and gain a concise overview of the issues.

Naturally with a subject of this type it is impossible to cover the issues from every angle. For example, as their role in healthcare increases due to the new information sources available to them, firsthand views of patients and consumers will be crucial to the development of this field. It would also have been relevant to explore the drivers involved in the purchase of and presumably self-determined compliance with over-the-counter medicines and also complementary and alternative medicines. However, these are evolving areas and the absence of quality published data somewhat restricts the conclusions that can be made. However, it is hoped that these areas can be addressed in the future.

Similarly, although a chapter exploring compliance issues in a silent disease area (cardiovascular disease) has been included, it would have been of interest to contrast this with compliance in the area of organ transplantation. Such a comparison could shed light on why patients fail to comply with their therapies, even in situations where failure to do so could be fatal. Once again, these issues can be explored in future editions of this book.

An introduction of this type would not be complete without an expression of our sincere gratitude to the contributing authors for their commitment and enthusiasm in labouring to cover such a vast field in such a concise manner. Equal thanks also go to the team at Gower – Jonathan Norman, Fiona Martin, Michael Dogwiler and Linda Cayford in particular – for their belief in us, their gentle support and unstinting enthusiasm for what we were so keen to achieve.

We were both very excited at the prospect of commissioning and editing a book on patient compliance as we both share a view that without compliance and concordance there is little point in healthcare interventions of any type. As Dr Jane Chin says in Chapter 9, 'Patient compliance is a multidimensional, multinational, and multidisease state problem'. We hope that this book will improve the understanding of readers on the key issues impacting on compliance as well as stimulate debate and discussion on how this important area can be further addressed for the future.

Dr Madhu Davies and Dr Faiz Kermani.
December 2005

Part 1
What is Compliance?

The opening chapters set the scene: they illustrate the scope of the issue, defining compliance, persistence, adherence and concordance together with the health economic impact of non-compliance and its consequent impact on public health.

CHAPTER 1

Patient Compliance: Setting the Scene

Dr Faiz Kermani and Dr Madhu Davies

Medical non-compliance is the failure of patients to comply with their medical care regimens. There is a host of health care professional– patient interactions which may be affected by non-compliance, ranging from medico-social issues such as patients refusing to accept 'Meals on Wheels'[1] when they are too frail to shop and/or cook for themselves, through to a conscious or unconscious decision, after going through all the trauma of an organ transplant, not to comply with anti-transplant rejection therapy.

In order to produce a manageable text for the reader, we have chosen to focus on the factors influencing compliance with medicines. We tried to obtain insights on compliance from the areas of complementary and alternative medicine and also consumer health but failed. We wanted to include these areas because patients often instigate the decision to access them without conventional healthcare professional intervention. By definition, they have engaged with the process, at least at the outset: what factors drive them to remain engaged and what factors turn them away from these options? We felt that there could be valuable lessons to learn and apply to conventional, mainstream medicine with its heavy reliance on pharmacology. We failed in our attempt because potential authors cited a lack of published data on which to base their chapters. We hope to address this problem in the next edition of this book.

So, from the perspective of this book, and very broadly, non-compliance refers to the failure of patients to take medicines in their prescribed manner. Where relevant, the authors set the scene for their topics and provide their working definitions of non-compliance; this in itself begins to illuminate the multi-faceted aspects of compliance.

---

1. Meals on Wheels: A United Kingdom intervention aimed at getting hot meals to those who need them in the community, typically the frail and elderly. A small charge is levied.

The problem of non-compliance is not a new one and it has been investigated for several decades worldwide. Regardless of the science and medical technology behind a particular drug, it will only be therapeutically effective if patients take it according to their doctors' recommendations.

Patient non-compliance with their medication lessens the quality of healthcare and, in some cases, can lead to dangerous consequences for patients. It is taken so seriously that the *New York Times* described the scale of its occurrence in the USA as the nation's 'other' drug problem (Zuger, 1998). It also has an important, and often underestimated, economic impact on healthcare. Now that the allocation of healthcare resources has become such an important issue for governments, healthcare providers can no longer ignore patient compliance issues. Some believe that advances in improving compliance may be as important as improving the actual treatments on offer.

The importance of patient compliance is also well recognized by those running clinical trials, as it has an important bearing on the evaluation of new drugs. Even though compliance in trials is often better than that seen in general clinical practice for many conditions, patient compliance is an important issue that must not be overlooked. For example, a Canadian study focusing on migraine concluded that better adherence to treatment could improve health outcomes, but that the compliance strategies available were mostly ineffective and were poorly assessed (Aubé, 2002). The therapeutic gain in many studies was, at best, in the order of 30–40 per cent, but the author suggested that the frequency of migraine attacks could be reduced by 50 per cent through effective compliance strategies (ibid.).

Paying attention to compliance issues is therefore essential to ensuring that the data collected during trials are as accurate as possible. When planning trials, clinical teams aim to ensure maximum patient compliance. Compliance will be affected by factors such as the duration of the treatment, the number of times a drug has to be taken per day and potential side-effects.

In mainstream medicine, prescribers, healthcare providers and manufacturers have struggled to determine the myriad factors that contribute to the non-compliance problem in order to counteract its effects. The field of compliance-related issues is growing, and there is considerable debate on the appropriate terminology to be used (Mullen, 1997). Much of the confusion has arisen from where the different terms to describe the usage of medicines have originated. Some terms and phrases are used exclusively in the clinical domain, some in the educational/social science arena and others in the pharmacoepidemiology/drug utilization research domain. Patient compliance remains a multi-faceted problem, and the difficulties in defining what is relevant to the field mean that there are no easy solutions.

Furthermore, as medical practice and social issues can vary widely around the world, approaches to improving patient compliance in one country cannot automatically be assumed to be appropriate for solving the problem in another. Internationally there will be variations in the preferences and dislikes of the patients in each individual nation or particular region. This means that all parties involved in healthcare must learn more about the societies from which these patients are drawn. It is sadly all too easy to make assumptions and generalizations about patients. Yet as we are only beginning to learn, patients' attitudes to their medicines can be influenced by many aspects of their daily life.

Understanding the patient's perspective on the disease in question can lead to considerable improvements in compliance. For example, a study on type I diabetes patients in England focused on the dietary constraints that the disease imposed ('Diabetics', 2002). The majority of these patients had to follow strict diets to ensure that their blood sugar levels remained stable. In the study, patients were divided into two groups. The first group were trained on how to adjust their insulin intake to take account of their changing diet, whereas the second group received their usual treatment. After six months, the researchers found that those in the first group had more stable blood sugar levels despite the fact that they were actually requiring more frequent insulin injections. The authors of the study concluded that that this approach would help patients 'to fit diabetes into their lives rather than their lives into diabetes'.

From a technical point of view, the nature of a medicine can affect patient compliance with a therapy. When developing a new drug, pharmaceutical companies often spend considerable time on assessing how the dosage form appropriate for their candidate will affect patient compliance. Consequently, novel drug delivery technologies are being applied to new drugs in the hope that they might encourage patients to comply with their treatment. Yet a form that proves popular in one country may not necessarily be as popular in another. However, unless those companies developing medicines communicate effectively with those who prescribe medicines and use them, few advances will be made in improving patient compliance.

These aspects of patient compliance are well known in the treatment of HIV infection with antiretroviral drugs. The antiretroviral therapies that are now available have the potential to achieve and sustain suppression of viral replication in many individuals, thereby transforming the outlook for patients. In many cases, HIV has been transformed into a manageable chronic disease (Altice and Fridland, 1998) provided that patients maintain a near-perfect adherence to therapy. However, studies have found that compliance rates vary substantially (ibid., Singh *et al.*, 1996), and it is well known that differing levels of adherence to therapy explain much of the magnitude and durability of the therapeutic response (Altice and Friedland, 1998).

Early on in the attempt to resolve this problem it was recognized that improving adherence was not the sole responsibility of the patient. As drug manufacturers and prescribers began to better understand patient attitudes to antiretrovirals, dramatic improvements were made in terms of compliance. Patients wished to take as few pills as possible and found the frequent dosing to be problematic (Dixon, 2002). Once-daily and twice-daily treatments have proved more acceptable to patients than those that had to be taken three times a day. Similarly, the use of fixed-dose combination antiretrovirals, which contain two or three antiretroviral drugs in a single formulation, can improve compliance. Reducing the number of pills and thereby reducing the frequency of dosage have enabled patients to fit the treatment in more easily with their lifestyles.

In this introductory chapter we have hopefully illustrated the range of factors that can affect patient compliance, all of which will be expanded upon and supplemented in the following chapters. As suggested above, in the modern context it is also important to appreciate that many patients are using complementary medicines based on their own assessment of their health. Compliance issues relating to these remedies have not been explored, but they could well have a bearing on how patients use the medicines prescribed by their physician.

As the field expands, it is hoped that there will be scope to widen the discussion concerning patient compliance further in the future.

REFERENCES

Altice, F.L. and Friedland, G.H. (1998), 'The Era of Adherence to HIV Therapy', *Annals of Internal Medicine*, **129**(6), pp. 503–505. Also available at: http://www.annals.org/cgi/content/full/129/6/503#R9-15.

Aubé, M. (2002), 'Improving Patient Compliance to Prophylactic Migraine Therapy', *Canadian Journal of Neurological Science*, **29**, Supplement 2, S40–S43.

'Diabetics "Freed from Strict Diets"' (2002), *BBC News*, 4 October at: http://news.bbc.co.uk/1/hi/health/2295325.stm.

Dixon, B. (2002), 'Reasons for Low Compliance with HAART Regimens Pinpointed', AIDSmeds.com at: http://www.aidsmeds.com/news/20021028publ005.html.

Mullen, P.D. (1997), 'Compliance Becomes Concordance', *British Medical Journal*, **314**, p. 691.

Singh, N., Squier, C., Sivek, C., Wagener, M., Nguyen, M.H. and Yu, V.L. (1996), 'Determinants of Compliance with Antiretroviral Therapy in Patients with Human Immunodeficiency Virus: Prospective Assessment with Implications for Enhancing Compliance', *AIDS Care*, **8**, pp. 261–69.

Zuger, A. (1998), 'The "Other" Drug Problem: Forgetting to Take Them', *New York Times*, 2 June.

CHAPTER 2

View from the Real World

Dr John Parkinson, Dr Li Wei and
Professor TM MacDonald

THE EXTENT AND EFFECT OF NON-COMPLIANCE

Poor adherence to treatment of chronic diseases is a worldwide problem of striking magnitude and adherence to long-term therapy for chronic illnesses in developed countries averages 50 per cent. In developing countries, the rates are even lower. It is undeniable that many patients experience difficulty following treatment recommendations.
(WHO, 2003)

Increasing the effectiveness of adherence interventions may have a far greater impact on the health of the population than any improvement in specific medical treatments.
(Haynes *et al.*, 2001)

The literature contains different terms that describe the phenomenon of 'compliance'. Already we have used two, compliance and adherence. We should therefore commence any discussion with a series of definitions of the various terms.

Definitions

Over the years, a whole series of words and phrases has been applied to the act of taking, or not taking, medicines 'as directed'. Some of these are used exclusively in the clinical domain, some in the educational/ social science area and others in the pharmacoepidemiology/drug utilization research domain. Care should be exercised as the use of these terms is not always consistent.

The variation in terms used can be partly explained by the different sources of drug use information, the precise type of data available or, sometimes, the tone of the message to be conveyed – particularly if work on behavioural science is being reviewed. The main words/phrases in current use, together with an explanation, follow.
Our intention here is not to dictate which definition is correct or should be used but to point out that anyone interested in the area should take care, when comparing results in different publications, to ensure that comparisons have meaning. Our own personal preferences for definitions will become clear later when we present research results.

Compliance

Compliance is the degree to which a patient is compliant with the instructions that are given by a healthcare professional and written on the medication label (for example, prescribed dose and time schedule). Accepting that compliance can involve both a time and dose dimension, it can be measured in a number of ways. These range from the absolute whereby there is some method of monitoring, using a biological marker, that the patient has actually swallowed or inhaled the medication, to pill counts that are often used in clinical trials, to a medication event monitoring system (MEMS) that records the date and time when a container was opened or activated, to electronic databases that record the redemption of a second or subsequent prescription of pills as a marker that the previous pills have been taken. In the latter case, the difference between the redemption dates should equal the number of days of medication available for 100 per cent compliance.

Some studies also report compliance rates as expressed by patients, but it has been noted that good compliers express this accurately whereas poor compliers tend to overstate their compliance (Cramer and Mattson, 1991; Spector *et al.*, 1986). There are also studies that report providers' recommendations, although these also tend to overestimate (Norell, 1981). The term 'compliance' is a value-laden and hierarchical term and, because of this, has been much criticized.

Adherence

Most authorities agree that adherence and compliance have the same meaning. However, a recent WHO report states that adherence requires the patient's agreement, thereby suggesting that compliance does not require this. The term 'adherence' is thus still authoritarian and has its critics (WHO, 2003). Others, including ourselves, have used adherence as a composite term to 'lump together' compliance and persistence.

For example, over a 100-day period a subject takes 56 tablets spread out evenly over these 100 days. The compliance is 56 per cent. Another subject takes 56 tablets on successive days and then stops. His persistence is 56 days. Another subject takes 56 tablets over 70 days and then none for 30 days. Over the first 70 days he is 80 per cent compliant but his persistence is only 70 days. However, over 100 days he is 56 per cent adherent. Thus adherence is a convenient term when examining the 'intention to treat' type of analyses of medicine use in large populations of subjects.

Non-adherence or non-compliance

Non-adherence or non-compliance is the degree to which patients do not comply or adhere to instructions. Indeed, some authors have gone further and defined degrees of non-compliance: non-compliance is less than 20 per cent compliance, partial compliance is 20–79 per cent and full compliance is 80 per cent or more (Insull, 1997).

Intelligent non-compliance

This term has been used to describe non-compliance that has been reasoned (on account of, say, feeling better, bad taste or side-effects) by a patient but might not necessarily be wise (Hindi-Alexander, 1987).

Primary non-compliance or non-redemption

This refers to the failure to redeem any of the medication prescribed, by failure to obtain the medications (Beardon *et al*, 1993). This can be at the level of failure to obtain all medications written on the prescription or failure to obtain some of them. This latter situation can occur where prescription charges or drug costs for all required drugs are higher than the patient can afford, with the consequence that the patient makes a decision to have just those that can be afforded. This decision may or may not be taken in conjunction with the dispenser.

Refill Compliance

This is, in the main, the most common measure of compliance/adherence of populations taking medications under real-world conditions. There can be various measures of refill compliance as measured using data from pharmacies about when patients collect medications measured in some way against the ideal of no gaps in therapy. Research studies using pharmacy-based data often just refer to adherence or compliance rates whilst others define this using the term 'refill compliance'.

Concordance

Caroline Kelham and her colleagues discuss concordance in more detail in Chapter 12. Concordance reflects the mutuality of the care process: the patient 'concords' with the view of his physician. This is a favoured term in the UK (see Marinker *et al.*, 1997). However, within concordance there remains the issue of what compliance or adherence rates ensue from the concordance activities.

Persistence/persistent

This term is used to describe the length of time a patient remains on a drug as calculated from pharmacy redemption data (see the discussion above on adherence). It is a useful indicator of how, in the real world, medications meet the needs of patients. Persistence has to be reviewed in the light of the length of any 'grace periods' that are allowed in a judgement of adherence that might otherwise suggest that persistence had ceased.

Grace period

A grace period is a specified time during which a patient, apparently, has no drug available, but may not be considered as non-adherent or non-persistent. Consider a patient who starts on a chronic medication and during the first 90 days consumes 90 tablets. Thereafter is a ten-day period when he does not renew his prescription. Is he 90 per cent adherent? Is he 100 per cent compliant for a period of 90 days and 0 per cent compliant for ten days? Or is he persistent for 90 days and 90 per cent adherent for 100 days? This example illustrates the differing ways in which such an observed behaviour pattern can be described. However, in interpreting the observed behaviour it is probable that the 'bathroom cabinet effect' comes into play. This effect occurs when subjects take medication imperfectly over time and are left with a residue at the end of any given period. There can then be a period of apparent complete non-compliance as they use up this residue. Thus most researchers require some 'grace period' when patients take no medication (as judged by some record of consumption) that has to be exceeded to determine the end of a period of use or 'persistence'. Often this is 45 or more days after the end of the last prescription.

Coverage

Coverage means that the patient has sufficient medication to take an adequate dose during the period concerned.

Medication possession ratio (MPR)

The MPR is the days of drug supplied/days of period. This is a specific measure of compliance that is often stated as a percentage.

The intrigue of compliance!

We will start with an intriguing and interesting study that also looked at compliance: The Coronary Drug Project (Coronary Drug Project Research Group, 1980) was a randomized double-blind clinical trial that compared clofibrate to a placebo, the outcome being mortality.

The study showed that good adherers to clofibrate – that is, patients who took 80 per cent or more of the protocol prescription during the five-year follow-up period – had a substantially lower five-year mortality rate than did poor adherers to clofibrate (15.0 versus 24.6 per cent; P = 0.00011). However, similar findings were noted in the placebo group – that is, 15.1 per cent mortality for good adherers and 28.3 per cent for poor adherers (P = 4.7 × 10–16). Thus patients who were better than 80 per cent adherent to the placebo had a 36 per cent reduced rate of death (RR=0.64) compared to those who were less than 80 per cent compliant to the placebo.

Is it credible that placebo affects mortality? Or was adherence in this study simply a surrogate marker for persons whose behaviour type predicts mortality? These findings show the serious difficulty, if not impossibility, of evaluating treatment efficacy in subgroups determined by patient responses (for example, adherence) after randomization.

As the reader of this chapter it might be informative to reflect on your own behaviour: can you honestly say that you have always complied fully with every tablet of every prescription and have always finished the course? A very few readers will say yes, with honesty. The reality is that nearly everyone is non-compliant; the variable is the degree of non-compliance.

Failure to take medications as instructed is an important problem in everyday clinical practice as, in many cases, the outcome expected will not be achieved (Wei *et al.*, 2002).

When looking at the issue from the point of one person taking one single drug once a day in the morning or twice a day, morning and evening, it can be hard to see why there is a problem. The reality is that most medications are taken in the later years of life for chronic conditions and often involve taking many different medications at varying intervals and at varying times; sometimes with the complication of some before food and some after. Even the rhythm of taking the small pink one in the morning with the red one and just the yellow one at night can be disrupted when, at the next collection of medications from the pharmacy, the small pink one becomes a different shade of yellow because the generic version rather than a branded version has been dispensed.

Figure 2.1 is a dramatic representation of real-world non-compliance. The data, spanning two years, are taken from a research study using our own Tayside dispensed prescribing database (Coronary Drug Project Research Group, 1980). Each column represents a person who has been prescribed a statin to lower his or her cholesterol level and, in so doing, reduce the overall cardiovascular risk. To gain full benefit from this treatment the medication must be taken continuously. Each line of squares represents a month's supply of treatment; if the square is white the person has picked up the prescription for the statin; if grey he or she has not and therefore could not have taken any medication that month. Black squares denote that no data were available after that month. The figure shows the following types of non-compliant behaviour:

1. early cessation without even change to an alternate treatment, subjects 10 and 11
2. occasional breaks in treatment (subject 16)
3. holidays from treatment, lasting a few months (subjects 2 and 4)
4. full compliance (subject 2)
5. sabbaticals from treatment lasting many months (subject 14).

The chart shows, for a range of subjects, whether or not they had statin medication, at the right dose, available in each month after being started on treatment. A white square shows that medication was available, a grey square that none was available. A black square denotes the end of the monitoring period of the study. Data has been shown for just two years.
Source: Coronary Drug Research Project Group (1980).

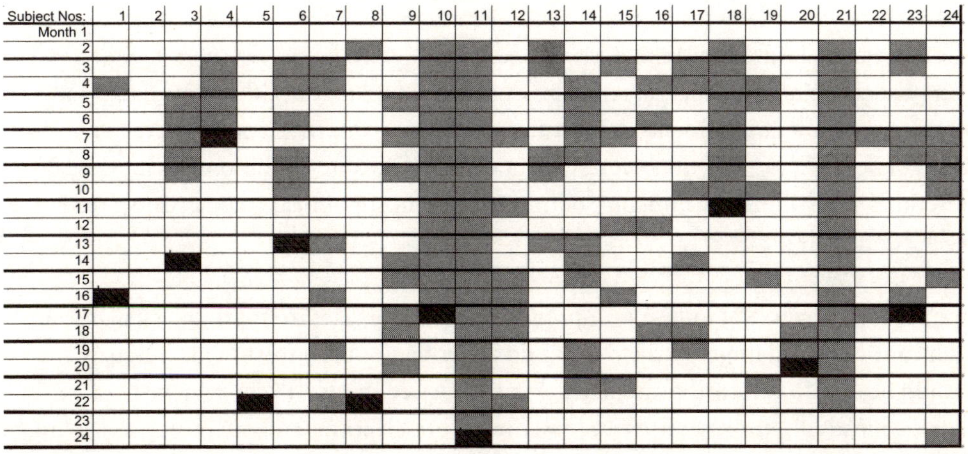

Figure 2.1 Patient compliance in taking statins over a two-year period

Analysis of all the data from the study showed that only about 1 in 100 people were 100 per cent compliant! The results of this research study will be reviewed later in this chapter.

In clinical studies that are used to provide the evidence base for drug treatment a great effort is made to select patients who have a single disease, are younger and are motivated and compliant. Within these trials extra resources are available to ensure that the subjects are as compliant as possible throughout the study period. These studies measure 'efficacy' in the 'ideal world' and are essentially measures only of drug behaviour. Efficacy data is important in order to ensure that, at a minimum, we know that a drug has some benefits that outweigh any risks of the treatment. But, within days of a new drug becoming widely available, it is being used by patients who differ, sometimes radically, from those in efficacy trials. They may be older or younger, have multiple co-morbidities, be taking many other medications, each requiring to be taken at different times and in different ways and have far less supportive care than is applied in the trial situation. In these circumstances what is measured by using routinely collected clinical (observational) retrospective data is 'effectiveness' – a measure of patient, doctor and drug behaviour as well as a measure of the 'organization of care'. Failure to take medications as directed is a major explanatory component in differences between efficacy and effectiveness.

Failure to take medications as directed also has considerable consequences for patients, providers and the pharmaceutical industry. Patients may get only partial or no benefit but potentially still have the risk of a drug-related adverse event. With acute treatments, such as antibiotics, they run the risk of treatment failure or antibiotic resistance thus limiting their own and society's armoury of useful antibiotics. With chronic treatments they may die earlier or suffer other more complicated medical conditions.

For providers, the outcomes of treatment are less than expected and, if models of chronic care delivery are not well constructed, they will fail to predict future healthcare needs and/or fail to show the improvement in health that is expected. In care delivery systems in which essentially all care (except prescription charges for some) is delivered free at the point of care, as in the UK, failure to comply leads to a considerable waste of limited NHS resources. On the other hand, the prospect of short-term drug budget escalation, if compliance were dramatically improved, does not enthral holders of the drug budget. Short-term goals often mean that many of the subsequent beneficial outcomes of good compliance are off the radar screen. This does not imply that healthcare professionals, civil servants and governments do not attempt to try to improve compliance; rather, that it might not be a top priority. Money spent now on chronic conditions for improved outcomes years ahead is a difficult political issue as most political goals are short term due to election cycles.

For the pharmaceutical industry, improved compliance leads to improved sales and additionally would improve the real-world effectiveness of its treatments. On paper, it should be easy to measure compliance, but in practice this is hard to achieve because, in many countries, information about prescribing, prescriptions and dispensing is not linked. This is exemplified by healthcare delivery in the UK whereby GPs do not have access to the information about whether a patient is even picking up any, some or all items on a prescription. This situation might possibly change with the advent of electronic prescribing and full interchange between doctor and pharmacy, but the current advice from the UK Information Commissioner on Data Protection is that such data can only be fed back from either the pharmacy where the prescription was encashed or from a central system if the patient has given explicit consent. This runs contrary to other sharing arrangements in the use of healthcare data where access is controlled on a need-to-know basis based on implicit consent.

Is compliance ever greater than 100 per cent?

Some subjects consume more drugs than prescribed, perhaps in the belief that more will be better. This is particularly true for drugs such as analgesics. However, the treatment of diabetes with insulin is an example of where the behaviour of some patients in their efforts to manage their condition leads them to 'consume' far more than they apparently need. Thus 'careful, fastidious' patients may keep insulin at home, at work (or school) and at other locations where they make regular visits. We will present data later showing this phenomenon.

However, before venturing further with the subject we need to establish a common understanding of the process from prescription to medication-taking.

THE PROCESS: PRESCRIPTION TO MEDICATION-TAKING

The exact process by which a patient obtains a prescription medication varies from country to country. The basic process is common as are the points at which the process can go wrong, leading to patients not taking their medication as directed.
The general process is as follows:

1. The *patient* visits the doctor.
2. The *doctor* makes a diagnosis.
3. The *doctor* discusses the diagnosis, illness, treatment and so on, and the *patient* accepts the advice (or not) and is given a drug or token to exchange for the drug.
4. The *patient* decides to accept that token and whether or not to get the medication.
5. The *pharmacist, doctor or other person* dispenses the drugs as on the prescription and provides advice (verbal and/or written) about taking the medication.

In some systems, including that of the UK, some patients may now be faced with a rationing decision; they cannot afford all the drugs they require and are forced to purchase only some of the medications at each pharmacy visit. The patient now has medication available but various factors will influence whether the patient takes the drug as directed. For the majority of patients it is a personal decision at each dose point to take their medication or not. The exceptions are children and those under the care of others (hospital or nursing home patients or those with care-givers at home). The factors that affect an intelligent decision at each dose point to take the medication or to reduce the dose, if tablets can be broken or the dose consists of more than one pill/tablet, are a decline in symptoms, a side-effect or, for non-symptomatic diseases, the fact that the patient may feel no different, leading to reduced use. Other causes may be confusion or forgetfulness, or a change of routine at weekends and the taking of an extended sleep or rest. There are also external reasons such as newspaper scare stories. Where a specific drug is involved the reason is obvious, but there may be knock-on effects about pill-taking in general. Finally, some people just do not like taking drugs!

At some point, just before the supply of the medication is exhausted the patient returns to a doctor to get a repeat prescription and may or may not be honest with the doctor about the missed doses/non-compliance. Alternatively, the patient uses some method, agreed with the prescriber, to obtain a repeat prescription.

In the processes described above it might seem that the important aspect is obtaining and taking the drug as prescribed. However, ultimately it is the outcome that is important. This might not always require that all doses of a drug are taken. Indeed, in short-term efficacy clinical trials patients who take 80 per cent or more of their medication, based upon pill counts, are usually considered 'compliant'.

For a chronic treatment taken over one year 80 per cent compliance is equivalent to missing 73 days of therapy or, in other words, only taking nine and a half months' therapy.

The fact that there may be a tolerance on what doses are taken to achieve the desired outcome is due to a series of factors that come into play between the taking of the medication, its activity and its excretion from the body. For each medication the pharmaceutical industry spends vast resources on ensuring that each drug is available in the right dose and at the right dose interval, which provides the correct steady state level of the drug at the site of its activity. Too high a level and there may be a risk of adverse events, too low a level and the effect of the drug will not be seen. This is a balance between the rates of absorption into the system, delivery to the site of action and the breakdown and excretion of the drug as researched in the population.

A population in which genetic differences, that we do not yet fully understand, create fast and slow metabolizers and excreters means that the ideal dose and interval may only be right for some. In choosing the dose and interval, reliance is placed on the difference between the dose that might cause an adverse reaction and one that is ineffective; the therapeutic window; it is wide.

Using pharmacokinetic and pharmacodynamic modelling and good drug design science, the chosen 'standard' dose and dose interval of modern drugs are designed to suit a large proportion of the population. However, this 'one size fits all' approach overlooks the considerable and unpredictable patient variability in compliance.

For some drugs, compliance has important societal implications. For example, vaccines taken widely can induce 'herd' immunity and, with tuberculosis, non-compliance can result in others being infected and the emergence of drug resistance. In the treatment of tuberculosis 'directly observed therapy' (DOT) has become the norm in patients who cannot reliably comply with treatment.

Much of the drug development and testing process takes place under ideal conditions that are not those seen in everyday clinical practice, with the consequence that patient compliance to a medication is often thought of in relation to the taking of one drug. In reality, many patients are taking multiple drugs to manage a single condition, hypertension being one such example. The elderly diabetic with osteoarthritis may well be taking five or six different medications daily – for life.

The taking of such a range of medications would be simplified if all could be taken at the same time and swallowed with the same liquid. In practice this rarely happens, and patients have to take medications at different times in the day, at different intervals and at varying times in relation to food. This recipe for unintentional non-compliance might perhaps be addressed by the concept of the 'polypill' – drugs that are regularly used together as individual drugs combined in one pill. This concept has been taken to the level of possibly including six drugs to 'reduce cardiovascular disease by more than 80 per cent' (Wald and Law, 2003). Interestingly, the authors of this article did not even make a comment on the effect that such a combination might have in improving outcomes via improvement in compliance. However, we need to be aware that failure to comply sufficiently with such a polypill might lead to worse overall outcomes than with poor compliance to only some of the individual drugs.

REAL-WORLD COMPLIANCE RESEARCH AND RESULTS

Quantitative research

To undertake compliance research it is necessary to have access to large population-based and well demographically described databases or record-linkable datasets that contain details of drug usage as well as the measure used to classify effectiveness. This might be hospitalizations, death or a laboratory measure of a surrogate marker of disease. In assessing the importance of any such research publication the strengths and weaknesses of the methodology used must be fully understood. For instance, drug data based on what a doctor prescribes, rather than on what a patient receives, does not take into account primary non-compliance (see later) and is also affected by the way in which primary care clinical information technology (IT) systems may be programmed to automatically produce repeat prescriptions at a set interval based on the previous prescription and providing the drug for the ideal 100 per cent compliance interval.

Examples of such quantitative research

Primary non-compliance and non-redemption (Hindi-Alexander, 1987)
Our research group has access to a dataset, unique to the UK, of dispensed medications – the ones actually picked up by the patient. We wanted to better understand the reasons for primary non-compliance and undertook a study comparing the written prescriptions with those actually dispensed by nine doctors over a three-month period. During the three-month period 2999 women (51 per cent) and 1855 men (33 per cent) received 13 457 and 7464 prescription items respectively. Of these patients14.5 per cent failed to redeem 1072 items (5.2 per cent). This failure to redeem was lowest in children and

increased with age. The highest rate of non-redemption was in women aged 16–29 and in men aged 40–49. Analysis by type of medication showed the highest non-redemption to be 38.6 per cent for oral contraceptives and that both men and women failed to redeem ear, nose and throat medications at the next highest level. Cardiovascular drugs and those for the eyes were redeemed at the highest rate. Prescriptions issued at weekends, usually given out by doctors attending patients out of hours, were the least likely to be redeemed despite the fact that intuitively these patients are most likely to want their symptoms reduced. Not surprisingly the lowest rate of non-redemption was amongst those exempt from paying any charge for each item on the prescription (see Figure 2.2). The prescriber influence on non-redemption was seen in the fact that prescriptions written by trainee doctors were least likely to be redeemed. Significant levels of non-redemption, as seen in this study, have subsequently been confirmed within the large UK general practice databases such as GPRD where there is only about 90 per cent concordance between the prescriptions issued by the GP and those recorded as being redeemed at a pharmacy by the UK Prescription Pricing Authority (Rodriguez *et al.*, 2000).

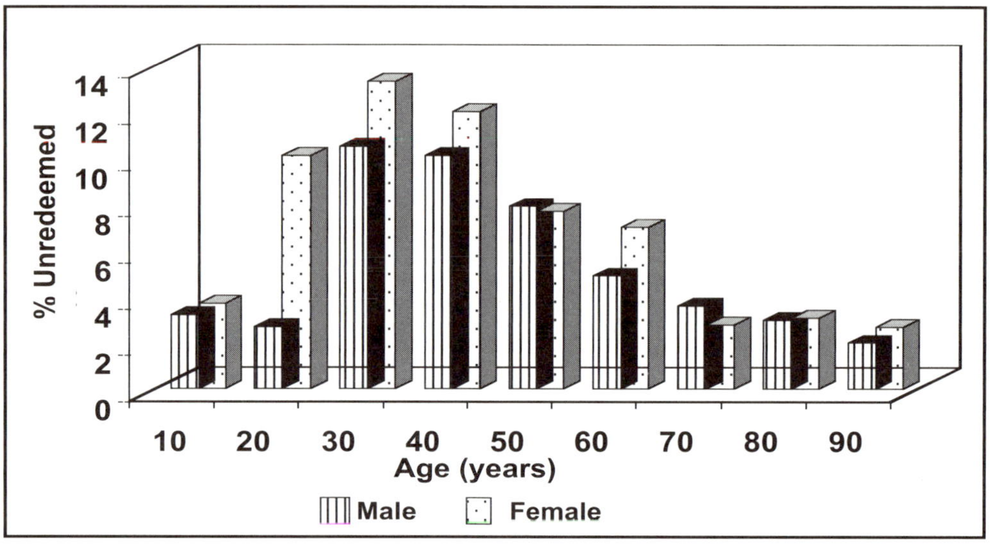

Figure 2.2 Percentage of patients failing to redeem their prescriptions, by age group and sex

The graph shows the percentage of patients, by sex, in each age group who failed to obtain their medications, having been given a prescription by their GP. The higher levels seen in the age range 18–60 are associated with the fact that this group are required, in the main, to pay a charge for each medicine on the prescription.
Source: MeMo data.

Compliance in type I diabetes (Morris et al.*, 1997)*
Adherence to insulin treatment in teenage type I diabetics is a serious matter, and clinical studies have shown that intensive treatment with insulin avoids both short- and long-term complications. It is therefore perhaps surprising that, in some patients, compliance to treatment is not only occasionally poor, but poor to the extent of patients missing

months of treatment! This study of adolescent subjects was conducted by linking the records of a population-based clinical care diabetes system (DARTS) with the dispensed prescribing dataset. The mean age of the subjects was 16 years with 51 per cent being male, the mean age at diagnosis was ten years and the mean duration of disease was seven years.

The difficulties of such compliance research had previously been pointed out, and this study was only possible because the medically recommended insulin dose was recorded for each person in the dataset and could be compared with the insulin actually redeemed to give an adherence index (maximum possible insulin coverage per year). In addition, measures of haemoglobin A1c (a measure of glycaemic control over the prior three months) and all hospitalization admissions were contained in the dataset. The hypothesis for the study was that poor glycaemic control was associated with failure to take insulin and that hospital admissions were related to non-adherence. The study included data from 89 subjects over the 18-month period from May 1993.

The results, illustrated in Figure 2.3, showed clearly the benefit of person-level data as the mean medically recommended insulin dose was 48 (19) IU per day but the collected insulin was 58 (25) IU per day, showing that, as a group, teenage diabetics collected and had more insulin available than was actually required. The mean insulin adherence index for the whole group was 486 days with the range being 119 days to 1060 days. However, 28 per cent of the subjects obtained less than the required 365 days' treatment and their mean was 250 days – over three months' missing insulin!
It was therefore not surprising that, of the ten patients admitted for diabetic ketoacidosis, nine had adherence indices below the required 365 days. The study showed that poor adherence was playing a large part in a phenomenon that had previously been thought to be more associated with insulin resistance secondary to pubertal hormone changes.

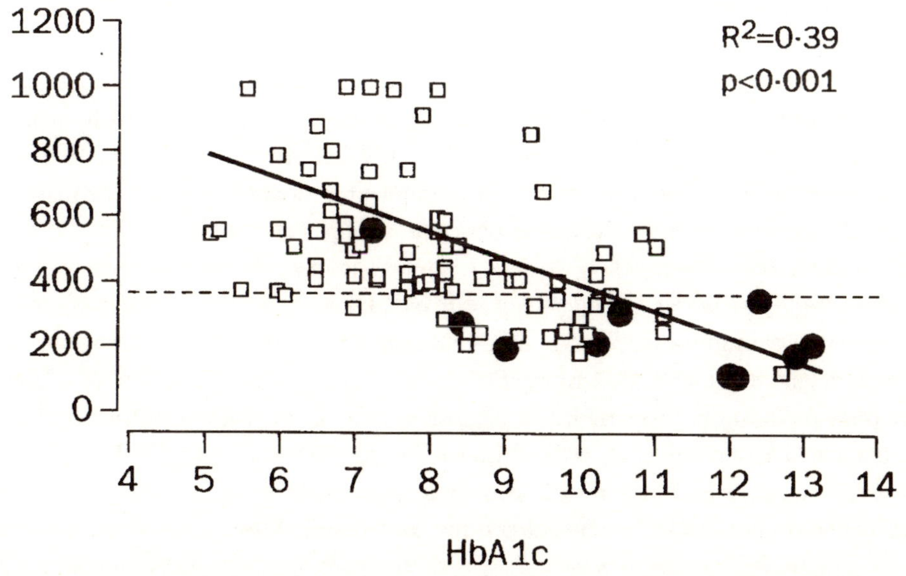

Figure 2.3 Compliance and non-compliance among teenage type I diabetic patients

HbA1c is a measure of glycaemic control. Black circles are subjects who were hospitalized for diabetic ketoacidosis. White squares are other subjects. The dotted line represents 365 days: levels of non-compliance are shown below the line; compliance greater than 100 per cent is shown above the line. *Source*: Morris *et al*. (1997)

Adherence to statin treatment and hospital readmission – the outcome measured (Coronary Drug Project Research Group, 1980)
Coronary heart disease is a leading cause of morbidity and mortality worldwide, and many large clinical trials (4S, CARE, WOSCOPS, LIPID, AFCAPS) have shown that statins reduce the risk of major coronary events by about 30 per cent. When considering improved survival in patients following a myocardial infarction (MI) or in high-risk primary prevention, it is important to understand how these results might translate into real-world treatment where adherence to treatment will be less than in the clinical studies. Other reports (for example, Sung *et al*., 1998) have suggested that only 37 per cent of participants take greater than 90 per cent of all doses of statins over a two-year period.

This study was carried out using the record-linkage database (MEMO) covering the 400 000 population of Tayside, Scotland that contains all dispensed community prescribing, hospital discharge data, biochemistry and other data linkable by a unique patient identifier. The study was a six-year follow-up study and tracked the course of 5590 patients who had experienced a myocardial infarction (MI). Comparison was made between those who received statin treatment and those that did not, as well as within the statin treated group looking at various levels of non-adherence to treatment.
The results showed that only those who had better than 80 per cent adherence had a significant reduction in their relative risk of MI and all-cause mortality compared with those receiving no treatment. The proportion of people on statins with better than 80 per cent compliance and who achieved a successful outcome was only 64 per cent.

Asthma: the use of the medication event monitoring system (MEMS) (Yeung et al.*, 1994)*
An interesting comparison was made in a clinical study of aerosol medication use in asthma. Patients were either made aware of the fact that a medication monitoring system enabled the doctors to know exactly when medication had been inhaled (actually when the device had been activated) or they were not told. When patients were aware of being monitored a majority (60 per cent) were fully compliant, but when unaware the majority had a compliance rate between 30 and 51 per cent (Yeung *et al*., 1994).

Transplantation: compliance with immunosuppressive medications
The availability of immunosuppressive drugs has enabled a range of transplant operations to take place with a reduced opportunity for rejection. It is obvious, however, that failure to take these medications properly has dire consequences for the patient. It has been estimated that lack of compliance is the third leading cause for rejection (Didlake *et al*., 1988). Other workers have reported 25 per cent non-compliance in a study covering 55 transplant centres with 1541 patients (Greenstein and Siegal, 1998).

The same workers reported three different types of lack of compliance: 'accidental non-compliers' (47 per cent), comprising those patients who sometimes forget to take the therapy; 'invulnerables' (28 per cent), comprising those patients who believe that they do not need to take their immunosuppressive drugs regularly; and 'decisive non-compliers' (25 per cent), comprising those patients who decide for themselves what therapy they should take.

Clinical monitoring research

How do we monitor compliance in individuals when we do not know whether they are collecting and consuming prescriptions? With some drugs, such as angiotensin-converting enzyme inhibitors (ACEIs), one can measure the direct effect in blood. ACEIs should result in serum ACE levels being near to zero. We have used this to monitor the consumption of ACEIs in subjects with congestive heart failure (Struthers *et al.*, 1999). Others have 'doped' medicines with low-dose phenobarbitone (Pullar *et al.*, 1991). This is a long-acting drug, and steady-state plasma levels in compliant subjects can be predicted for any individual. Other approaches include the actual measurement of the drug within the plasma – a measure often used in epilepsy when seizure control is lost. In hypertension where blood pressure control is poor despite multiple drug therapy a supervised trial of directly observed dosing is often useful. Patients are asked to attend a day ward having not taken their tablets that morning. An automated sphygmomanometer is set to monitor blood pressure every 15 minutes or so, and they sit quietly in a chair until stable baseline readings are obtained. They are then given their prescribed medication. Some subjects have dramatic blood pressure responses to this, some becoming hypertensive. These patients are likely to be non-compliant. In other patients the blood pressure does not change much. These have truly resistant hypertension.

INTERVENTIONS TO IMPROVE COMPLIANCE

A recent review of interventions to improve adherence to medication prescriptions concluded that current methods are mostly complex, labour-intensive and not predictably effective (MacDonald *et al.*, 2002). Much work is required to understand, measure and more effectively develop effective interventions in this behaviourally complex condition. It is our belief that such research is vital if we are going to make a significant impact on the outcomes of drug treatment in those with poor adherence to prescription drugs.

CONCLUSION: THE FUTURE

Much pharmacoepidemiology and drug utilization research still needs to be undertaken if we are to fully understand real-world effectiveness. Furthermore, the data used to support such research should also be available to healthcare professionals to help them improve compliance.

A number of pharmaceutical companies have started extensive patient compliance programmes for their drugs. This is laudable if such schemes work, but the results of such efforts need to be fully researched not only on the drug concerned, but also on all the other medications that the patient is taking. If compliance for all could be improved we would applaud this.

However, it might just be that improved compliance on one drug, taken in one manner, has a negative effect on the compliance of other drugs. We do not know and we need to find out!

Devices to help medication compliance are already available but will no doubt become more technically advanced. As we know, however, advances come at a cost – a cost that many health providers would find hard to swallow! Devices also cover the use of mobile phones and SMS text messaging that potentially offer a cheap method of aiding compliance – we carry them everywhere. The current situation in which the elderly have the lowest use of mobile phones is only a short-term issue.

The era of personalized medicines is on the radar screen and this will offer patients the drug that is right and effective for them and will cause them the fewest adverse reactions. In the concordance era it would seem that such an offering will enable the doctor–patient interaction to be more positive than at present – a change from 'this drug might help you' to 'this drug will help you' and to 'this drug is unlikely to cause you the tolerance problems you have previously experienced'. This fact alone should have a major impact on people's willingness to take a drug as directed.

REFERENCES

Beardon, P.H.G. *et al.* (1993), 'Primary Non-compliance with Prescribed Medication in Primary Care', *British Medical Journal*, **307**, pp. 846–48.

Coronary Drug Project Research Group (1980), 'Influence of Adherence to Treatment and Response of Cholesterol on Mortality in the Coronary Drug Project', *New England Journal of Medicine*, **303**, pp. 1038-41.

Cramer, J.A. and Mattson, R.H. (1991), 'Monitoring Compliance with Antiepileptic Drug Therapy', in J.A. Cramer, and B. Spilker (eds), *Patient Compliance in Medical Practice and Clinical Trials*, New York: Raven Press, pp. 123–37.

Didlake, R.H., Dreyfus, K., Kerman, R.H. *et al.* (1988), 'Patient Noncompliance: A Major Cause of Late Graft Failure in Cyclosporine-treated Renal Transplants', *Transplantation Proceedings*, **20**, pp. 63–69.

Garcia Rodriguez, L.A., Perez-Gutthann, S. and Jick, S. (2000), 'The UK General Practice Research Database', in B.L. Strom (ed.), *Pharmacoepidemiology* (3rd edn), Chichester: Wiley, pp. 375–85.

Greenstein, S.M. and Siegal, B.R. (1998), 'Compliance and Noncompliance in Patients with a Functioning Renal Transplant: A Multicenter Study', *Transplantation*, **66**, pp. 1718–26.

Haynes, R.B. *et al.* (2001), 'Interventions for Helping Patients to Follow Prescriptions for Medications', *Cochrane Database of Systematic Reviews*, Issue 1. Now superseded by Issue 2 (2006).

Hindi-Alexander, M. (1987), 'Compliance or Noncompliance: That is the Question!', *American Journal of Health Promotion*, **1**, pp. 5–11.

Insull, W. (1997), 'The Problem of Compliance to Cholesterol Lowering Therapy', *Journal of Internal Medicine*, **241**, pp. 317–25.

MacDonald, H.P., Garg, A.X. and Haynes, R.B. (2002), 'Interventions to Enhance Patient Adherence to Medication Prescriptions', *Journal of the American Medical Association*, **288**, pp. 2868–79.

McNabb, W.L. (1997), 'Adherence in Diabetes: Can We Define It and Can We Measure It?', *Diabetes Care*, **29**, pp. 215–28.

Marinker, M., Blenkinsopp, A., Bond, C., Briten, N., Feely, M., George, C. et al. (eds) (1997), *From Compliance to Concordance: Achieving Shared Goals in Medicine Taking*, London: Royal Pharmaceutical Society of Great Britain.

Morris, A.D. et al. (1997), 'Adherence to Insulin Treatment, Glycaemic Control and Ketoacidosis in Insulin-Dependent Diabetes Mellitus', *The Lancet*, **350**, pp. 1505–10.

Norell, S.E. (1981), 'Accuracy of Patient Interviews and Estimates by Clinical Staff in Determining Medication Compliance', *Social Science and Medicine – Part E, Medical Psychology*, **15**, pp. 57–61.

Pullar, T., Kumar, S., Chrystyn, H., Rice, P., Peaker, S. and Feely, M. (1991), 'The Prediction of Steady-state Plasma Phenobarbitone Concentrations (Following Low-dose Phenobarbitone) to Refine its Use as an Indicator of Compliance', *British Journal of Clinical Pharmacology*, **32**(3), pp. 329–33.

Spector, S.L. *et al*.(1986), 'Compliance of Patients with Asthma with an Experimental Aerosolized Medication: Implications for Controlled Clinical Trials', *Journal of Allergy and Clinical Immunology*, **77**, pp. 65–70.

Struthers A D., Anderson, G., MacFadyen, R. J., Fraser, C. and MacDonald, T. M. (1999), 'Non-adherence with ACE Inhibitor Treatment is Common in Heart Failure and Can be Detected by Routine Serum ACE Activity Assays', *Heart*, **82**, pp. 584–88.

Sung, J.C., Nichol, M.B., Venturini, F. *et al.* (1998), 'Factors Affecting Patient Compliance with Antihypertensive Medications in an HMO Population', *American Journal of Managed Care*, **4,** pp. 1421–30.

Wei, L. *et al.* (2002), 'Adherence to Statin Treatment and Readmission of Patients after Myocardial Infarction: A Six Year Follow up Study', *Heart*, **88**(3), pp. 229–33.

Wald, N.J. and Law, M.R. (2003), 'A Strategy to Reduce Cardiovascular Disease by More than 80 Per Cent', *British Medical Journal*, **326**, pp. 1419–24.

WHO (2003), 'Adherence to Long-term Therapies: Evidence for Action', July at: http://www.who.int/chronic_conditions/adherencereport/en/index.html (accessed July 2005).

Yeung, M. *et al.* (1994), 'Compliance with Prescribed Drug Therapy in Asthma', *Respiratory Medicine*, **88**, pp. 31–35.

CHAPTER 3

Health Economic Aspects of Patient Non-Compliance

Dr Dyffrig Hughes

Economics is concerned with the allocation of resources in a world where resources are finite and demands are potentially infinite. Health economics, a subdiscipline of economics, focuses on the allocation of healthcare resources within the context of resource scarcity. Health economic evaluations are a set of tools used to assess the efficiency, or value for money, of health technologies. They require that both costs and health benefits are assessed to determine whether incremental health gains justify the costs. Cost-effectiveness analyses allow medicines that produce a common unidimensional health benefit, such as life-years gained or symptom-free days, to be compared. Cost–utility analyses, where outcomes are measured in terms of quality-adjusted life-years (QALYs), allow economic considerations to be made across a wide range of interventions. In cost–benefit analyses, attempts are made to value all the relevant costs and benefits in monetary terms.

There are many aspects of non-compliance that need to be considered within an economic framework. First is the importance of considering non-compliance in economic evaluations and the related differences between efficacy and effectiveness. Second is the impact of non-compliance on healthcare costs and efficiency (cost-effectiveness) of drug treatments. The final aspect is the assessment of the cost-effectiveness of interventions aimed at improving compliance. This chapter will focus on the first two issues.

INCORPORATING NON-COMPLIANCE IN ECONOMIC EVALUATIONS

The majority of economic evaluations rely on evidence on health outcomes from randomized controlled trials (RCTs). Such trials, which are often conducted for regulatory purposes, address issues of efficacy and not necessarily clinical effectiveness. Clinical effectiveness refers to how drugs perform in routine use as opposed to in controlled trials that are often highly selective in their inclusion criteria. It is not uncommon for trials to exclude patients who are non-compliant during the run-in phase in order to increase the probability that treatment is successful (Pablos-Mendez *et al.*, 1998). Although this is satisfactory for the requirements of regulatory authorities, it is less so when decisions on resource allocation need to be made. In such circumstances, 'real-world' outcomes are considered to be more relevant and appropriate (Bombardier and Maetzel, 1999; Revicki and Frank, 1999). This section addresses issues concerned with clinical effectiveness, as opposed to efficacy, and how these relate to pharmacoeconomic evaluations and the cost-effectiveness of drug treatments.

Therapeutic efficacy is best determined from the results of RCTs in which the test drug is compared to placebo or standard therapy. These maximize internal validity by limiting confounding factors and biases through randomization and blinding such that observed differences can be causally ascribed to different treatments. Although allocation biases may be eliminated in RCTs, a concern that is frequently expressed is whether or not patients who are recruited and subsequently selected for inclusion in RCTs are a true representation of the population to which the drug is to be made available. Differences may arise when generalizing from RCTs to real-world situations of drug therapy (Rothwell, 1995; Tonkin, 1998).

Patients are most often recruited to trials from atypical institutions such as teaching hospitals by enthusiastic and experienced practitioners who bear little resemblance to the majority of doctors (Black, 1996). Once recruited, the run-in phase of the RCT specifically weeds out 'inappropriate' patients for reasons such as non-response or non-compliance (Pablos-Mendez *et al.*, 1998).Thereafter, eligible patients are randomized to treatment only if consent is granted. Thus the structure of RCTs is such that the patients selected for investigation are homogenous and unlikely to be truly representative of the patient population at large (Rothwell, 1995; Tonkin, 1998).

For some drugs, differences between efficacy and effectiveness are pronounced (Bombardier and Maetzel, 1999; Revicki and Frank, 1999). These are attributable, in part, to differences in compliance – and, in particular, persistence. When considering these differences, it is useful to distinguish between the two main forms of non-compliance:

1. *Drug regimen non-compliance.* This is to do with how patients take their tablets. How many doses are missed? What are the variations in the timing of doses? What is the frequency of 'drug holidays' (a phenomenon where patients effectively take a break from taking their tablets for three or more days)?

2. *Premature discontinuation of drug therapy*. This is arguably the most important form of non-compliance to consider – in particular for chronic therapies of asymptomatic diseases (such as hypercholesterolaemia). It is measured as the proportion of patients who discontinue therapy after one year, two years and so on.

For chronic diseases there are instances where persistence in routine practice is as low as 13 per cent over five years (Catalan and LeLorier, 2000), compared with between 69 per cent and 94 per cent (over five to seven years of treatment) in RCTs of lipid-lowering therapies (Insull, 1997). Clearly, in such circumstances the clinical benefits (efficacy) reported in RCTs will not be achieved in a substantial proportion of patients.

It is important to recognize the various reasons why non-compliance may, or may not, result in differences between efficacy and effectiveness. These are largely related to drug and disease attributes, although they are clearly dependent on differences in compliance and persistence between trial and non-trial participants.

Significant compliance-related differences may exist between efficacy and effectiveness in situations where:

- compliance in routine practice is much worse than in clinical trials (for instance, if cost is a cause of non-compliance in routine practice, or if non-compliant patients were excluded during the trial run-in phase)
- the drug is very unforgiving, and therefore missing one or two doses may be critical. Forgiveness is a measure of the ability of a drug to maintain therapeutic activity despite the presence of non-compliance (Urquhart, 1996).
- drugs have a very narrow therapeutic window. These require careful dosing regimens and punctual remedication, which may be achieved in controlled trials, but not in routine practice.
- the dosing regimen is incorrect. Examples might include drugs that are prescribed on a once-daily basis, with the intention of improving compliance, even though they should in fact be prescribed twice daily at half-dose.

Small or no differences may exist between efficacy and effectiveness in cases where:

- patients are equally as good, or bad, at complying in routine practice as they are in clinical trials
- the drug is very forgiving, and therefore the desired therapeutic effect is still maintained despite doses being missed
- the drug is highly effective, in which case it may not matter whether all doses are taken or not, as it will still work
- the study design used to compare efficacy and effectiveness is inadequately powered to show equivalence between efficacy and effectiveness – absence of evidence is not the same as evidence of absence
- the prescribed dose is incorrect. This is more common than might be expected (Heerdinck *et al*., 2002; Cross *et al*., 2002). Larger doses than required are likely to elicit responses on the plateau of the dose–response relationship, and therefore non-compliance will effectively be equivalent to a leftward shift along the dose–response curve, but still within a region where pharmacological responses are beneficial.

CASE STUDY: LIPID-LOWERING AGENTS

The importance of considering compliance when assessing clinical and cost effectiveness will be illustrated using lipid-lowering drugs as a case study. Cardiovascular diseases pose a high burden, both in terms of health impact and healthcare costs. There is extensive evidence to support the effectiveness of HMG-CoA reductase inhibitors (statins), particularly in reducing morbidity and mortality related to cardiovascular disease (LaRossa *et al.*, 1999). There is also evidence to suggest that differences may exist between outcomes observed in clinical trials and in routine practice. One study, for instance, suggested that the ratio of observed to expected reduction in low-density lipoprotein (LDL) cholesterol with statins is 0.75 ±0.69 for pravastatin, 0.79 ±0.48 for atorvastatin and 0.88 ±0.61 for simvastatin.

Several studies have assessed compliance with lipid-lowering agents, most of which have focused on statin therapy. The review that follows is not intended to be a systematic account of all such studies, but serves to illustrate the disparity that exists between intended continuous therapy and the prevalence of non-compliance that exists in routine practice (Hughes and Bagust, 2001).

Drug regimen non-compliance

A subgroup analysis of the Expanded Clinical Evaluation of Lovastatin (EXCEL) study was performed by Shear *et al.* (1992). Percentage changes from baseline in LDL cholesterol levels were obtained from 7721 moderately hypercholesterolaemic patients (>4.14 mmol/l) taking a range of doses of lovastatin. Compliance was assessed by self-reporting, and expressed as the percentage of study days in which patients took tablets. The positive association between compliance and decrease in LDL cholesterol is evident in the figures presented in Table 3.1.

Table 3.1 The association between compliance and LDL cholesterol (% change from baseline ± SEM) according to treatment group

	Compliance category		
Intervention group	80%	90%	100%
Placebo	+0.6 (0.3)	–2.9 (0.9)	–6.3 (1.8)
Lovastatin 20mg daily	–24.6 (0.3)	–19.5 (0.8)	–14.5 (1.5)
Lovastatin 40mg daily	–31.1 (0.3)	–26.6 (0.8)	–22.1 (1.5)
Lovastatin 20mg twice daily	–34.2 (0.3)	–29.7 (0.7)	–25.1 (1.5)
Lovastatin 40mg twice daily	–41.3 (0.3)	–34.0 (0.8)	–26.6 (1.6)

Source: Shear *et al.* (1992).

In a subgroup analysis of the West of Scotland Coronary Prevention Study (WOSCOPS, 1997), patients taking more than 75 per cent of doses experienced a 32 per cent risk reduction for all-cause mortality. This compared with a 22 per cent reduction in non-compliers. Compliance was assessed as the relative frequency of visits at which trial medication was issued. The figures relating to the analysis, presented in Table 3.2, indicate that compliance is a major contributory factor for the difference in mortality risk.

Table 3.2 The association between compliance and relative risk reduction (95 per cent confidence interval) for pravastatin versus placebo for coronary heart disease death or non-fatal MI, cardiovascular death and all-cause deaths, as reported in the WOSCOPS trial

	Compliance category		
Outcome	<75%	75–100%	100%
Coronary heart disease death or non-fatal MI	1.01 (0.66, 1.54)	0.61 (0.37, 0.99)	0.62 (0.49, 0.78)
Cardiovascular death	0.80 (0.38, 1.68)	0.45 (0.19, 1.06)	0.72 (0.46, 1.13)
All death	1.01 (0.66, 1.54)	0.71 (0.45, 1.12)	0.68 (0.45, 1.02)

Source: WOSCOPS Study Group (1997).

Bruckert *et al.* (1999) conducted an open-label trial to study the nature of non-compliance with fluvastatin in 4813 patients with primary hypercholesterolaemia over one year. One arm of the trial included patients who received information normally given by practitioners, and therefore was considered to reflect normal practice. The other arm consisted of patients who were better informed about the therapy. A total of 2888 subjects (75 per cent) were defined as compliant (taking more than 90 per cent of the prescription) and 957 (25 per cent) non-compliant. Although no attempt was made to relate these findings to changes in LDL cholesterol, in the non-compliant group there were a larger number of symptomatic patients who thought that the drug did not improve symptoms.

More reliable evidence relating to drug regimen non-compliance comes from studies that have monitored dosing patterns with an electronic event monitor (Urquhart, 1997). Tablet counts do not adequately capture the subtleties of drug-regimen non-compliance (Pullar *et al.*, 1989). Schwed *et al.*, (1999) monitored the dosing behaviour of 40 hypercholesterolaemic patients taking fluvastatin in normal clinical practice over a period of six months. Compliance with the total prescribed dose was 89 per cent, compared with 93 per cent as assessed by tablet count: 38 per cent of patients took drug holidays, and 9 per cent omitted doses for seven or more days (extended drug holidays). Almost half of the patients took more than one prescribed dose daily. Patients with a compliance to the total prescribed dose of less than 80 per cent experienced a 18 ± 18 per cent decrease in LDL cholesterol, compared with 22 ± 9 per cent for the range 80–90 per cent compliance and 24 ± 10 per cent for those who complied with greater than 90 per cent of total prescribed dose.

Premature discontinuation

Oster *et al.* (1996) reported a one-year discontinuation rate of 28 per cent with lovastatin 20mg daily in a US trial that was designed to approximate typical practice. Similar discontinuation rates were reported by Andrade *et al.* (1995) who conducted a retrospective cohort study based on the medical records of new users of lovastatin. Of 537 courses of lovastatin therapy, the one-year risk of discontinuing therapy was 15 per cent. The authors also reviewed other studies that evaluated discontinuation rates for lovastatin and noted that, in RCTs, the risk of discontinuation at six months ranged from 2.5 per cent to 10 per cent, compared with 3.6 per cent to 21.1 per cent in open-label trials.

A large population-based study of over 7000 patients that monitored persistence with statins was reported by Avorn *et al.* (1998). Patients failed to fill prescriptions for 35.7 per cent of the year. After five years, about 50 per cent had stopped using lipid-lowering therapy altogether.

Simons *et al.* (1996) evaluated the apparent discontinuation rates in 610 patients who were newly prescribed lipid-lowering drugs. Discontinuation, which was calculated as the proportion of patients who failed to collect prescription refills, was 60 per cent after one year. Half of the discontinuations occurred within three months and a quarter within one month of starting treatment.

The one-year and four-year discontinuation rates for statins from another observational study of 970 patients taking lipid-lowering therapy, were reported to be 10 per cent and 28 per cent respectively (Hiatt *et al.*, 1999). This compared with 48 per cent and 71 per cent for patients taking niacin, and 59 per cent and 83 per cent for patients on bile acid sequestrants.

Eriksson *et al.* (1998) assessed persistence with pravastatin in a Swedish primary care setting. Of 528 and 521 patients receiving 20mg and 40mg daily doses respectively, 403 (76 per cent) and 409 (78 per cent) completed the two-year study. For those who persisted with the lower dose, LDL cholesterol reduced from 5.55 $\pm$0.04 mmol/l at baseline to 4.08 $\pm$0.04 mmol/l after two years. This contrasted with a reduction from 5.45 $\pm$0.07 mmol/l at baseline to 5.14 $\pm$0.11 mmol/l over the same period in those who discontinued.

Strandberg *et al.* (1997) looked at the changes in cholesterol levels and patient compliance one year after the end of the Scandinavian Simvastatin Survival Trial (4S), by means of a questionnaire survey of 785 surviving 4S participants. The authors found that 74 per cent of patients had used cholesterol-lowering drugs after the study and 63 per cent were still using them (mostly simvastatin). The reported mean serum cholesterol levels were 5.1 $\pm$ 1.0 and 5.7 $\pm$1.1 mmol/l in current and non-users, respectively.

By far the least favourable persistence rates were reported in a Canadian study by Catalan and Lelorier (2000). In a cohort of subsidized, new users of statins, patients of similar ages to those in the WOSCOPS trial continued with therapy for a median of 173 days (95 per cent confidence intervals – CI 155, 204). Only 13 per cent of patients persisted for five years of treatment.

Discontinuation rates vary from study to study. One-year persistence ranges from 90 per cent down to 40 per cent (Oster *et al.*, 1996; Andrade *et al.*, 1995; Avorn *et al.*, 1998). However, the rate of discontinuation appears to decrease in subsequent years such that, after five years, persistence is in the region of 45 per cent and 13 per cent (Catalan and LeLorier, 2000; Larsen *et al.*, 2002). In patients who fail to persist, LDL cholesterol and other clinical endpoints are consistently less favourable than in patients who comply.

Taken together, the studies suggest that compliance appears to be relatively high in patients who possess statins, with the majority taking 90 per cent of prescribed doses over a six-month to one-year time period (Bruckert *et al.*, 1999; Schwed *et al.*, 1999). For these patients, the impact of drug-regimen non-compliance on lipid profiles depends on the extent to which statins forgive to non-compliance or, in other words, how critical it is to remedicate punctually. There is no direct evidence on this, but, for lovastatin, a significant compliance-dependency is apparent (Shear *et al.*, 1992). Increasing compliance from 80 per cent to 100 per cent is associated with a further 10 per cent reduction in LDL cholesterol, suggesting that lovastatin may not be as forgiving as other statins. There may be differences among statins in their ability to forgive to non-compliant dosing behaviour, and this may be related to their durations of action; the greater the duration of action in relation to the dosing interval, the more forgiving the drug (Urquhart, 1996). A simulation study of atorvastatin corroborates this theory, as its extended duration of action renders it forgiving to dose-regimen non-compliance (Hughes and Walley, 2003).

Of more relevance is the impact this may have on clinical endpoints such as coronary events and survival, particularly as mechanisms independent of LDL lowering may also play an important role in the clinical benefits conferred by these drugs. In patients who withdraw prematurely from statin treatment there is strong evidence to suggest that unfavourable cardiac events are more likely to occur (Heeschen *et al.*, 2002: Wei *et al.*, 2002). The analysis of the WOSCOPS study confirms that the relative risk reduction in cardiac and all-cause mortality is greatest for pravastatin when compliance is high (WOSCOPS Study Group, 1997).

The implications of the differences between efficacy and effectiveness are that cost-effectiveness estimates based on RCT data that ignore non-compliance – and persistence in particular – are likely to be biased. Such are the consequences of poor compliance that establishing its economic impact should be an integral part of any pharmacoeconomic evaluation. Failure to do so may lead to biased cost-effectiveness estimates and incorrect decisions on the allocation of healthcare resources. Figure 3.1, which presents a schematic representation of the cost-effectiveness plane, illustrates how decreasing effectiveness may render a drug cost-ineffective. The section that follows will explore this in more detail and will look, in particular, at the empirical evidence on the impact of non-compliance on healthcare costs and cost-effectiveness. Where available, evidence on whether non-compliance affects the decision on whether or not a treatment is cost-effective will be presented.

If it is assumed that healthcare systems are willing to afford £30 000 per additional QALY, then under conditions of full compliance, the drug is regarded as cost-effective and will be reimbursed. If non-compliance results in reduced benefits and increased healthcare costs, then the drug becomes

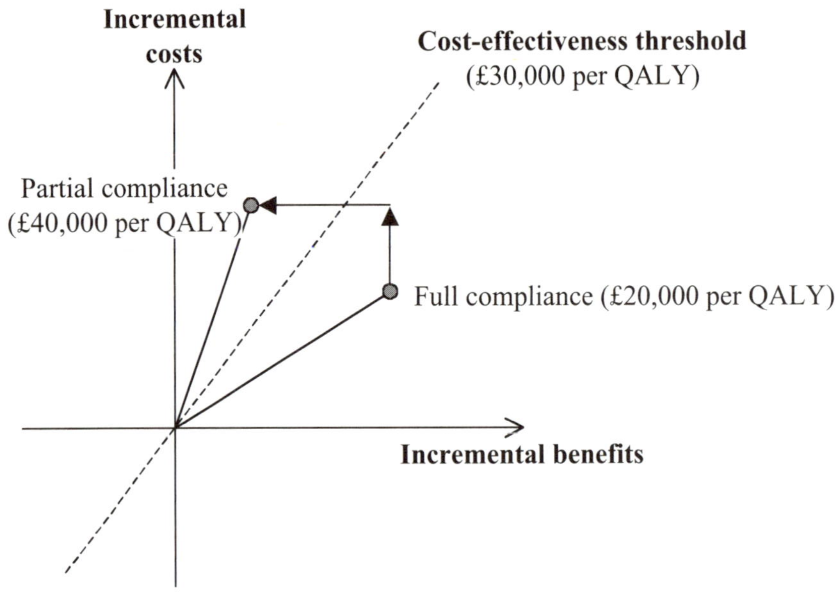

Figure 3.1 Schematic representation of the cost-effectiveness plane, whereby incremental costs are plotted against the incremental benefits

cost-ineffective at £40 000 per additional QALY, reducing the chances of it being adopted by publicly-funded healthcare systems.

THE IMPACT OF NON-COMPLIANCE ON HEALTHCARE COSTS AND COST-EFFECTIVENESS

The clinical and economic consequences of non-compliance depend on a number of factors, including the type and pattern of non-compliance, the extent of drug forgiveness, the degree of drug effectiveness, whether the drug alleviates symptoms or affects the progression of the disease, the severity and chronicity of the disease and whether or not rebound or withdrawal effects may develop (Hughes, 2002: Hughes *et al.*, 2001a; Cleemput and Kesteloot, 2002). For drugs that are potentially life-saving, non-compliance may have profound negative effects. For instance, non-compliance with immunosuppressants among transplant patients may result in tissue rejection which is not only associated with impaired quality of life, but also may necessitate expensive remedial surgery (Dobbels *et al.*, 2004). By contrast, for expensive but often ineffective treatments (for example, beta interferon in unresponsive patients with multiple sclerosis), non-compliance in terms of failure to redeem prescriptions may prove to be cost-saving without having a significant impact on disease progression or symptoms (Hughes *et al.*, 2001b).

A review by Peterson and McGhan (2005) examined the pharmacoeconomic impact of non-compliance with statins. They identified only two relevant studies and commented that many other studies discussed medication non-compliance as a factor, but did not independently analyse this in the pharmacoeconomic analysis. The first study, by

Urquhart (1999) described the pharmacoeconomic impact of variable compliance in patients taking non-statin lipid-lowering agents. A linear relationship between compliance and relative reduction in coronary artery disease risk was observed. The cost of preventing one coronary event over one year of treatment in a European healthcare system increased from US$180 810 with full compliance (numbers needed to prevent one cardiovascular event, NNT = 210) to US$651 777 (NNT = 757) with low compliance. By contrast, a small decline was observed in a UK, US or Canadian healthcare setting, from US$180 810 to $162 755 for the corresponding levels of compliance. In the European setting, prescriptions are often linked to follow-up visits and consequently sufficient quantities of drug are dispensed to last until the next visit – at times up to six months' supply. In the UK, USA or Canada, one or two months' supply of medications is more typically dispensed.

In the second study, Peterson and his colleagues (2002) analysed a US database of 2317 patients to determine the short-term (≤ 1 year) impact of non-compliance with statin medications. Their analysis showed that compliance (measured as medication possession ratio) was weakly correlated with total medical costs ($r=0.114$, $p<0.0001$). Similarly, there was a smaller, but statistically significant, relationship between compliance and total direct medical costs ($r=0.05$, $p=0.01$).

A recent retrospective cohort study (Sokol *et al.*, 2005) evaluated the impact of medication non-compliance on healthcare utilization and costs for hypercholesterolaemia, diabetes, hypertension and congestive heart failure in 137 277 patients in the USA. Non-compliance was defined as the number of days' supply of maintenance medications, obtained from administration claims data, for each condition. For hypercholesterolaemia and diabetes, high levels of compliance were associated with lower disease-related medical costs. Higher medication costs were more than offset by medical cost reductions, producing an overall reduction in healthcare costs. For hypertension, medical costs tended to be lowest at 80–100 per cent compliance, but differences were generally not statistically significant. Differences for congestive heart failure were also not significant.

Increases in the risk of hospitalization, defined as the probability of one or more hospitalizations during a 12-month period, were evident in all four conditions as compliance levels declined (Sokol *et al.*, 2005). Diabetic patients in the 80–100 per cent compliance group had a 13 per cent risk of diabetes-related hospitalization, compared with 20 per cent in the 60–79 per cent group, and 24 per cent in the 40–59 per cent compliance group. Similarly, for hypertensive patients, high levels of compliance (80–100 per cent) were associated with a reduced risk of hypertension-related hospitalization (19 per cent) compared to lower levels of compliance (40–59 per cent, 24 per cent risk). When considering all-cause hospitalization, a more pronounced difference was apparent, possibly indicating that non-compliance with one medication is associated with non-compliance with other medications for co-morbid conditions.

In a study of similar design, using insurance claims as a measure of medication compliance in 57 687 diabetic patients, Hepke *et al.* (2004) noted that increased compliance was associated with decreased medical care costs. However, increased compliance was not associated with decreased overall healthcare costs because medication costs offset medical care cost savings.

Tu *et al.* (2005) presented a novel study that compared intended and projected (based on compliance patterns) mean plasma concentrations of metoprolol for patients with heart failure. It was shown, by use of pharmacokinetic modelling, that deviations from intended concentrations were associated with increased numbers of emergency department visits and hospital admissions. Thus, for metoprolol, the maintenance of adequate plasma drug concentrations,achieved by patients compliant with the dosing instructions results in improved outcomes and reduced healthcare utilization.

A review of pharmacoeconomic evaluations which considered compliance was conducted by Hughes *et al.* (2001b). Besides the clear absence of consideration of compliance in the evaluation of pharmaceuticals (only 22 studies were identified from a database of 3000 health economic evaluations[1]), they also noted inadequacies in the reporting of non-compliance, invalid assumptions relating to the health outcomes and costs associated with poor compliance, and problems in the way in which health economists model the impact of poor compliance.

Most of the studies identified were of treatments for chronic diseases – only two (Genç and Mårdh, 1997; Scott and Alexander, 1998) considered drug regimen non-compliance with acute diseases. Generally speaking, the definitions given for non-compliance were inadequate. This has particular implications as a definition of the percentage of patients complying with a drug regimen (Clark *et al.*, 2000; Taylor *et al.*, 1997; Glazer and Ereshefsky, 1996; Fiscella and Franks, 1996), for example, provides no useful information as this may include drug regimen compliance or persistence, or both. In two cases (Vakil and Fennerty, 1996; Haddix *et al.*, 1995) the authors made no attempt at defining their measure of compliance. Some studies (Clark *et al.*, 2000; Taylor *et al.*, 1997; Brown *et al.*, 1997; Revicki *et al.*, 1997) defined an arbitrary proportion of doses taken, below which patients were considered to be non-compliant.

Similar inadequacy existed for the source of compliance rates used in the evaluations. Whilst most evaluations referred to compliance rates from relevant clinical studies (Clark *et al.*, 2000; Taylor *et al.*, 1997; Fiscella and Franks, 1996; Haddix *et al.*, 1995; Golan *et al.*, 1999; Lafata *et al.*, 2000; Rosner *et al.*, 1998; Rocchi and Tingey, 1997; Wasley *et al.*, 1997), or used base-case compliance rates derived from the results of individual clinical trials (Moore and Chaisson, 1997; Brown *et al.*, 1996; Brown *et al.*, 1999; Kobelt *et al.*, 1998; Lapierre *et al.*, 1995), the remainder used values based on assumptions or on medical opinion (Genç and Mårdh, 1997; Scott and Alexander, 1998; Glazer and Ereshefsky, 1996; Vakil and Fennerty, 1996; Brown *et al.*, 1997; Revicki *et al.*, 1997) or did not state the source of compliance data (Plans-Rubio, 1998; Garton *et al.*, 1997). Only five studies used a range of compliance levels in the sensitivity analysis which were

1. These studies were: Genç and Mårdh (1997); Scott and Alexander (1998); Clark *et al.*(2000); Taylor *et al.* (1997); Glazer and Ereshefsky (1996); Fiscella and Franks (1996); Vakil and Fennerty (1996); Haddix *et al.* (1995); Brown *et al.* (1997); Revicki *et al.* (1997); Golan *et al.* (1999); Lafata *et al.* (2000); Rosner *et al.* (1998); Rocchi and Tingey (1997); Wasley *et al.* (1997); Moore and Chaisson (1997); Brown *et al.* (1996); Brown *et al.* (1999); Kobelt *et al.* (1998); Lapierre *et al.* 1995); Plans-Rubio (1998); and Garton *et al.* (1997).

based on clinical evidence (Brown *et al.*, 1997; Lafata *et al.*, 2000; Rocchi and Tingey, 1997; Wasley *et al.*, 1997; Moore and Chaisson, 1997). The remainder used arbitrarily chosen compliance levels.

Although many evaluations made references to changes in risk probabilities or outcomes under conditions of non-compliance, only four made reference to evidence-based sources of clinical success rates (Clark *et al.*, 2000; Taylor *et al.*, 1997; Glazer and Ereshefsky, 1996; Lafata *et al.*, 2000). The majority either relied on assumptions based on opinion or did not disclose the source of clinical evidence. In some instances, authors provided no indication of the differences in health benefits that would be observed when patients were non-compliant (Fiscella and Franks, 1996; Haddix *et al.*, 1995; Plans-Rubio, 1998). No study directly measured the costs of non-compliance. Rather, deviations in costs were calculated by modelling the changes in resource utilization which would result from the observed (or assumed) alterations in therapeutic response.

A common approach adopted was to consider patients as either being compliers or non-compliers by defining an arbitrary proportion of doses taken – below which patients were categorized as non-compliers (Clark *et al.*, 2000; Taylor *et al.*, 1997; Brown *et al.*, 1997; Revicki *et al.*, 1999). Those who were 'non-compliers' experienced different event rates and outcomes from compliers. For example, one study (Taylor *et al.*, 1997) assumed the compliance rate to be the proportion of patients taking at least 60 per cent of their [*H. pylori* eradication] medications. Non-compliers were defined as experiencing 77 per cent of the eradication success rate of the compliers. All the studies which took non-compliance as meaning the proportion of patients discontinuing treatment per unit of time assumed that non-compliers experienced the same risk as untreated patients. In these studies, with the exception of one (Golan *et al.*, 1999), a constant annual rate of discontinuation was assumed.

From the studies evaluated, the direction and magnitude of the change in costs and consequences resulting from applying sensitivity analysis to the compliance rate was measured and taken as an indicator of the impact of non-compliance. There was consistency among studies, in that as compliance decreased (whatever the measure), the benefits also decreased. This is illustrated in Figure 3.2, where the percentage changes in outcome, corresponding to the compliance levels considered in the sensitivity analysis of each study, are plotted on a common set of axes. There is no consistency, however, in the direction of change in costs resulting from changes in compliance (which is shown in the same manner in Figure 3.3). Whilst some studies show that costs increase as compliance decreases, others showed the opposite trend. This difference did not appear to be related to the nature of the disease, the measure of non-compliance or the assumptions relating to the health benefits experienced by non-compliers. One study (Clark *et al.*, 2000) showed an initial decrease in cost as the compliance rate decreased, followed by an increase at lower levels of compliance.

A more recent study that incorporated persistence into the economic assessment of drugs for urinary incontinence (Hughes and Dubois, 2004) showed that assumptions relating to patients who discontinued therapy prematurely significantly influenced the cost-effectiveness of the drugs. With the assumption of full persistence (equivalent to clinical

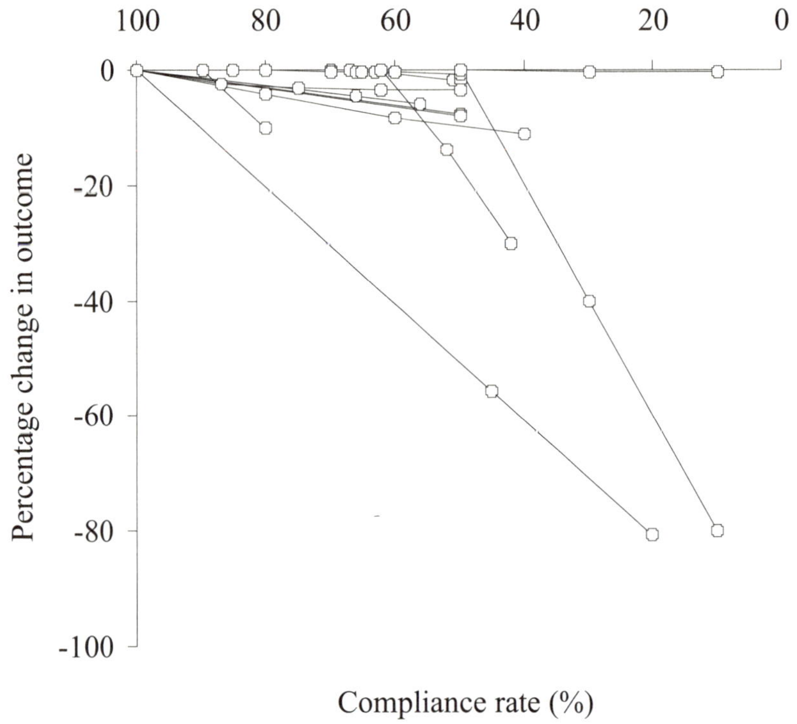

Figure 3.2 A plot of the percentage change in outcome in relation to compliance levels (both drug-regimen and discontinuation)

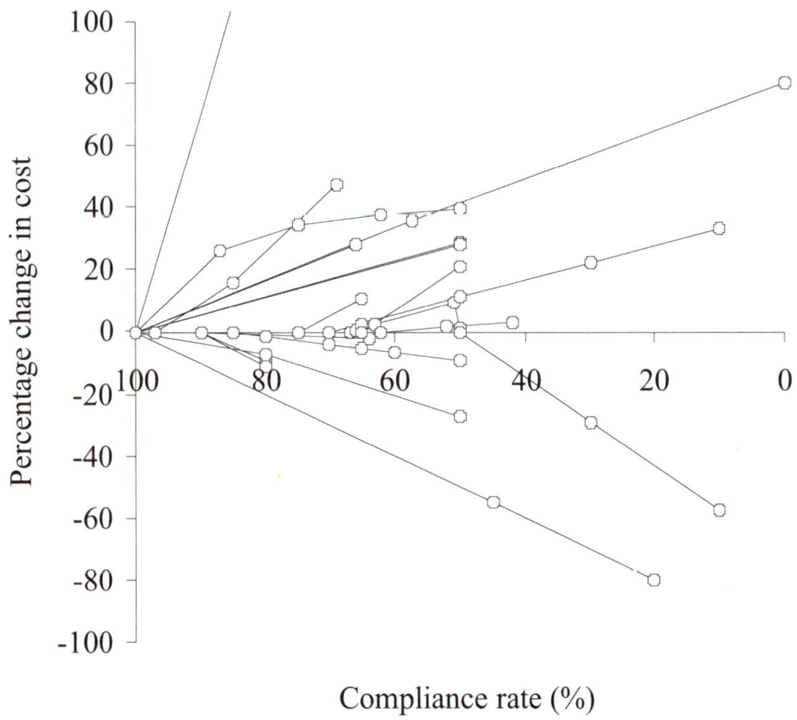

Figure 3.3 A plot of the percentage change in cost in relation to compliance levels (both drug-regimen and discontinuation)

trial setting), the short-acting formulation of oxybutynin was shown to be most cost-effective, at £5.81 per incontinent-free week. The long-acting formulation of oxybutynin, as well as two formulations of tolterodine, were more effective than immediate-release oxybutynin but at additional costs per incontinence-free week. In routine practice, however, six-month persistence with drugs for urinary incontinence is as low as 10 per cent. The base-case analysis of the evaluation assumed that patients discontinued either as a consequence of experiencing side-effects, in which case they reverted to baseline characteristics, or that they experienced some health benefit and decide not to continue with therapy. These patients were assumed to experience the same benefits as patients in the placebo group. The cost per incontinent-free week for the short-acting formulation of oxybutynin was calculated as £5.81. The incremental cost per incontinence-free week for the long-acting formulations of tolterodine and oxybutynin was £7.14 and £84.82, respectively.

The economic evaluations described demonstrate that medical expenditures do not always increase because of poor compliance. However, the limitations in the methodology adopted in many of the studies would suggest that the reported changes in healthcare expenditure may not necessarily be observed in practice. It is difficult, therefore, to predict the true economic impact of non-compliance with drug therapy, particularly as evidence relating to discontinuers is often not reported. It is the case, however, that decisions on optimal treatments, based on economic criteria, are influenced by non-compliance, in particular where factors listed on p. 25 are applicable.

A review of the economic impact of non-compliance by Cleemput *et al.* (2002), identified five studies that examined both the costs and consequences of non-compliance in economic evaluations. Two were cost–benefit analyses. The study by Rizzo *et al.* (1996) assessed the labour productivity effects of prescribed medicines for chronically ill workers. In the case of hypertension, increasing compliance with prescribed medication was estimated to reduce absenteeism by up to 2.05 days. The resulting net benefit was calculated to be US$169 per patient. Eastaugh and Hatcher (1982) assessed the efficacy of a triage process, whereby patients were subdivided into groups that were more predisposed to benefit from a given health education approach. The total annual cost saving in earnings loss per hypertensive patient in the control group versus the compliance-enhancing intervention group was US$26. The cost–benefit ratio of different interventions ranged from 1.24 to 2.2, indicating that benefits of the triage method for achieving medication compliance clearly outweigh its costs.

The three cost-effectiveness analyses identified by Cleemput *et al.* (2002) included an analysis of compliance-enhancing interventions with malaria prophylaxis, a cost-effectiveness analysis of medication and inhaler compliance intervention in asthma, and an evaluation of compliance intervention in outpatient geriatric patients. These studies focused more on the economics of compliance-enhancing interventions than on the economic impact of non-compliance. A more recent review of such studies was conducted by Elliott *et al.* (2005).

CONCLUSIONS

Health economic evaluations often fail to include non-compliance with medications. As a significant proportion of evaluations are based on efficacy trials, attention should be given to how their findings might be generalized. In particular, as poor compliance is one of the most important elements responsible for the differences that may exist between the effectiveness and efficacy of an intervention, greater consideration should be given to compliance when generalizing from the results of a controlled clinical trial. An optimal cost-effective treatment strategy chosen on the basis of efficacy data may not be so attractive once real-world compliance figures are taken into account.

Furthermore, the impact of non-compliance on both health benefits and healthcare resource utilization is potentially considerable. Measures to contain costs and improve outcomes need to be evaluated. These may include programmes to improve compliance, which should be assessed in terms of their cost-effectiveness according to standard methodology. It may be that for treatments effective against serious conditions, where non-compliance significantly affects operational effectiveness, targeted programmes to improve compliance may be an appropriate and cost-effective use of healthcare resources.

REFERENCES

Andrade, S.E., Walker, A.M., Gottlieb, L.K., Hollenberg, N.K., Testa, M.A., Saperia, G.M. and Platt, R. (1995), 'Discontinuation of Antihyperlipidemic Drugs – Do Rates Reported in Clinical Trials Reflect Rates in Primary Care Settings?', *New England Journal of Medicine*, **332**, pp. 1125–31.

Avorn, J., Monette, J., Lacour, A., Bohn, R.L., Monane, M., Mogun, H. and LeLorier, J. (1998), 'Persistence of Use of Lipid-lowering Medications: A Cross-national Study', *Journal of the American Medical Association*, **279**(18), pp. 1458–62.

Black, N. (1996), 'Why We Need Observational Studies to Evaluate the Effectiveness of Health Care', *British Medical Journal*, **312**(7040), pp. 1215–18.

Bombardier, C. and Maetzel, A. (1999), 'Pharmacoeconomic Evaluation of New Treatments: Efficacy versus Effectiveness Studies?', *Annals of the Rheumatic Diseases*, **58**, Suppl. 1, pp. 182–85.

Brown, M.C.J., Nimmerrichter, A.A. and Guest, J.F. (1999), 'Cost-effectiveness of Mirtazapine Compared to Amitriptyline and Fluoxetine in the Treatment of Moderate and Severe Depression in Austria', *European Psychiatry*, **14**, pp. 230–44.

Brown, M.G., Murray, T.J., Fisk, J.D., Sketris, I.S., Schwartz, C.E. and LeBlanc, J.C. (1996), *A Therapeutic and Economic Assessment of Betaseron in Multiple Sclerosis*, Ottawa, Canada: Canadian Coordinating Office for Health Technology Assessment.

Brown, R.E., Kendall, M.J., Halpern, M.T. (1997), 'Cost Analysis of Once-daily ISMN versus Twice-daily ISMN or Transdermal Patch for Nitrate Prophylaxis', *Journal of Clinical Pharmacological Therapy*, **22**, pp. 67–76.

Bruckert, E., Simonetta, C. and Giral, P. (1999), 'Compliance with Fluvastatin Treatment Characterization of the Non-compliance Population within a Population of 3845 Patients with Hyperlipidemia. CREOLE Study Team', *Journal of Clinical Epidemiology*, **52**, pp. 589–94.

Catalan, V.S. and LeLorier, J. (2000), 'Predictors of Long-term Persistence on Statins in a Subsidized Clinical Population', *Value Health*, **3**, pp. 417-26.
Clark, W.F., Churchill, D.N., Forwell, L., Macdonald, G. and Foster, S. (2000), 'To Pay or Not to Pay? A Decision and Cost-utility Analysis of Angiotensin-Converting-Enzyme Inhibitor Therapy for Diabetic Nephropathy', *Canadian Medical Association Journal*, **162**, pp. 195–98.
Cleemput, I. and Kesteloot, K. (2002), 'Economic Implications of Non-compliance in Health Care', *Lancet*, **359**(9324), pp. 2129–30.
Cleemput, I., Kesteloot, K. and DeGeest, S. (2002), 'A Review of the Literature on the Economics of Noncompliance. Room for Methodological Improvement', *Health Policy*, **59**(1), pp. 65–94.
Cross, J., Lee, H., Westelinck, A., Nelson, J., Grudzinskas, C. and Peck, C. (2002), 'Postmarketing Drug Dosage Changes of 499 FDA-approved New Molecular Entities, 1980–1999', *Pharmacoepidemiology and Drug Safety*, **11**(6), pp. 439–46.
Dobbels, F., De Geest, S., van Cleemput, J., Droogne, W. and Vanhaecke, J. (2004), 'Effect of Late Medication Non-compliance on Outcome after Heart Transplantation: A 5-year Follow-up', *Journal of Heart and Lung Transplantation*, **23**(11), pp. 1245–51.
Eastaugh, S.R. and Hatcher, M.E. (1982), 'Improving Compliance among Hypertensives: A Triage Criterion with Cost–Benefit Implications', *Medical Care*, **20**(10), pp. 1001–17.
Elliott, R.A., Barber, N. and Horne, R. (2005), 'Cost-effectiveness of Adherence-Enhancing Interventions: A Quality Assessment of the Evidence', *The Annals of Pharmacotherapy*, **39**(3), pp. 508–15.
Eriksson, M., Hadell, K., Holme, I., Walldius, G. and Kjellstrom, T. (1998), 'Compliance with and Efficacy of Treatment with Pravastatin and Cholestyramine: A Randomized Study on Lipid-lowering in Primary Care', *Journal of Internal Medicine*, **243**, pp. 373–80.
Fiscella, K. and Franks, P. (1996), 'Cost-effectiveness of the Transdermal Nicotine Patch as an Adjunct to Physicians' Smoking Cessation Counselling', *Journal of the American Medical Association*, **275**, pp. 1247–51.
Frolkis, J.P., Pearce, G.L., Nambi, V., Minor, S. and Sprecher, D.L. (2002), 'Statins do not Meet Expectations for Lowering Low-density Lipoprotein Cholesterol Levels When Used in Clinical Practice', *American Journal of Medicine*, **113**, pp. 625–29.
Garton, M.J., Cooper, C. and Reid, D. (1997), 'Perimenopausal Bone Density Screening – Will it Help Prevent Osteoporosis?', *Maturitas*, **26**, pp. 35–43.
Genç, M. and Mårdh, P-A. (1997), 'Cost-effective Treatment of Uncomplicated Gonorrhoea Including Co-infection with Chlamydia Trachomatis', *Pharmacoeconomics*, **12**, pp. 374–83.
Glazer, W.M. and Ereshefsky, L. (1996), A Pharmacoeconomic Model of Outpatient Antipsychotic Therapy in 'Revolving Door' Schizophrenic Patients', *Journal of Clinical Psychiatry*, **57**, pp. 337–45.
Golan, L., Birkmeyer, J.D. and Welch, H.G. (1999), 'The Cost-effectiveness of Treating All Patients with Type 2 Diabetes with Angiotensin-converting Enzyme Inhibitors', *Annals of Internal Medicine*, **131**, pp. 707–08.
Haddix, A.C., Hillis, S.D. and Kassler, W.J. (1995), 'The Cost Effectiveness of Azithromycin for Chlamydia Trachomatis Infections in Women', *Sexually Transmitted Diseases*, **22**, pp. 274–80.

Heerdink, E.R., Urquhart, J. and Leufkens, H.G. (2002), 'Changes in Prescribed Drug Doses After Market Introduction', *Pharmacoepidemiology and Drug Safety*, **11**(6), pp. 447–53.

Heeschen, C., Hamm, C.W., Laufs, U., Bohm, M., Snapinn, S. and White, H.D. (2002), 'Withdrawal of Statins Increases Event Rates in Patients with Acute Coronary Syndromes', *Circulation*, **105**, pp. 1446–52.

Hepke, K.L., Martus, M.T. and Share, D.A. (2004), 'Costs and Utilization Associated with Pharmaceutical Adherence in a Diabetic Population', *The American Journal of Managed Care*, **10**(2), Pt 2, pp. 144–51.

Hiatt, J.G., Shamsie, S.G. and Schectman, G. (1999), 'Discontinuation Rates of Cholesterol-lowering Medications: Implications for Primary Care', *The American Journal of Managed Care*, **5**, pp. 437–44.

Hughes, D.A. (2002), 'Economic Impact of Poor Compliance with Pharmaceuticals', *Expert Reviews in Pharmacoeconomics & Outcomes Research*, **2**, pp. 89–97.

Hughes, D.A. and Bagust, A. (2001), 'Impact of Non-compliance on the Cost-effectiveness of Statin Therapy', *Value in Health*, **4**(6), p. 489.

Hughes D.A. and Dubois, D. (2004), 'Cost-effectiveness Analysis of Extended-release Formulations of Oxybutynin and Tolterodine for the Management of Urge Incontinence', *Pharmacoeconomics*, **22**(16), pp. 1047–59.

Hughes, D.A. and Walley, T. (2003), 'Predicting "Real World" Effectiveness by Integrating Adherence with Pharmacodynamic Modeling', *Clinical Pharmacology and Therapeutics*, **74**(1), pp. 1–8.

Hughes, D.A., Bagust, A., Haycox, A. and Walley, T. (2001a), 'Accounting for Noncompliance in Pharmacoeconomic Evaluations', *Pharmacoeconomics*, **19**(12), pp. 1185–97.

Hughes, D.A., Bagust, A., Haycox, A. and Walley, T. (2001b), 'The Impact of Non-compliance on the Cost-effectiveness of Pharmaceuticals: A Review of the Literature', *Health Economics*, **10**, pp. 601–15.

Insull, W. (1997), 'The Problem of Compliance to Cholesterol Altering Therapy', *Journal of Internal Medicine*, **241**(4), pp. 317–25.

Kobelt G., Jonsson, L. and Mattiasson, A. (1998), 'Cost-effectiveness of New Treatments for Overactive Bladder: The Example of Tolterodine, a New Muscarinic Agent: A Markov Model', *Neurourology and Urodynamics*, **17**, pp. 599–611.

Lafata, J.E., Martin, S.A., Kaatz, S. and Ward, R.E. (2000), 'The Cost-effectiveness of Different Management Strategies for Patients on Chronic Warfarin Therapy', *Journal of General Internal Medicine*, **15**, pp. 31–37.

Lapierre, Y., Bentkover, J., Schainbaum, S. and Manners, S. (1995), 'Direct Cost of Depression: Analysis of Treatment Costs of Paroxetine versus Imipramine in Canada', *Canadian Journal of Psychiatry*, **40**, pp. 370–37.

LaRossa, J.C., He, J. and Vupputuri, S. (1999), 'Effects of Statins on Risk of Coronary Disease: A Meta-analysis of Randomized Controlled Trials', *Journal of the American Medical Association*, **282**, pp. 2340–46.

Larsen, J., Andersen, M., Kragstrup, J. and Gram, L.F. (2002), 'High Persistence of Statin Use in a Danish Population: Compliance Study 1993–1998', *British Journal of Clinical Pharmacology*, **53**, pp. 375–78.

Moore, R.D. and Chaisson, R.E. (1997), 'Cost Utility Analysis of Prophylactic Treatment with Oral Ganciclovir for Cytomegalovirus Retinitis', *Journal of Acquired Immune Deficiency Syndromes and Human Retrovirology*, **16**, pp. 15–21.

Oster, G., Borok, G.M., Menzin, J., Heyse, J.F., Epstein, R.S., Quinn, V., Benson, V., Dudl, R.J. and Epstein, A.M. (1996), 'Cholesterol-reduction Intervention Study (CRIS): A Randomized Trial to Assess Effectiveness and Costs in Clinical Practice', *Archives of Internal Medicine*, **156**, pp. 731–79.

Pablos-Mendez, A., Barr, R.G. and Shea, S. (1998), 'Run-in Periods in Randomized Trials: Implications for the Application of Results in Clinical Practice', *Journal of the American Medical Association*, **279**(3), pp. 222–25.

Peterson, A.M. and McGhan, W.F. (2005), 'Pharmacoeconomic Impact of Non-compliance with Statins', *Pharmacoeconomics*, **23**(1), pp. 13–25.

Peterson, A.M., Sanoski, C. and McGhan, W.F. (2002), 'Total Direct Medical and Drug Costs of Non-adherence to Statin Therapy within the First Year of Treatment: International Society for Pharmacoeconomics and Outcomes Research [abstract]', *Value in Health*, **3**, p. 167.

Plans-Rubio, P. (1998), 'Cost-effectiveness Analysis of Treatments to Reduce Cholesterol Levels, Blood Pressure and Smoking for the Prevention of Coronary Heart Disease; Evaluative Study Carried out in Spain', *Pharmacoeconomics*, **13**, pp. 623–43.

Pullar, T., Kumar, S., Tindall, H. and Feely, M. (1989), 'Time to Stop Counting the Tablets?', *Clinical Pharmacology and Therapeutics*, **46**(2), pp. 163–68.

Revicki, D.A. and Frank, L. (1999), 'Pharmacoeconomic Evaluation in the Real World. Effectiveness versus Efficacy Studies', *Pharmacoeconomics*, **15**(5), pp. 423–34.

Revicki, D.A., Brown, R.E., Keller, M.B., Gonzales, J., Culpepper, L. and Hales, R.E. (1997), 'Cost-effectiveness of Newer Antidepressants Compared with Tricyclic Antidepressants in Managed Care Settings', *Journal of Clinical Psychiatry*, **58**, pp. 47–58.

Rizzo, J.A., Abbott, T.A. III and Pashko, S. (1996), 'Labour Productivity Effects of Prescribed Medicines for Chronically Ill Workers', *Health Economics*, **5**(3), pp. 249–65.

Rocchi, A. and Tingey, D. (1997), 'Economic Evaluation of Dorzolamide vs. Pilocarpine for Primary Open-angle Glaucoma', *Canadian Journal of Ophthalmology*, **32**, pp. 414–18.

Rosner, A.J., Grima, D.T., Torrance, G.W., Bradley, C., Adachi, J.D., Sebaldt, R.J. and Willison, D.J. (1998), 'Cost Effectiveness of Multi-therapy Treatment Strategies in the Prevention of Vertebral Fractures in Postmenopausal Women with Osteoporosis', *Pharmacoeconomics*, **14**, pp. 559–73.

Rothwell, P.M. (1995), 'Can Overall Results of Clinical Trials be Applied to all Patients?', *Lancet*, **345**(8965), pp. 1616–19.

Schwed, A., Fallab, C.L., Burnier, M., Waeber, B., Kappenberger, L., Burnand, B. and Darioli, R. (1999), 'Electronic Monitoring of Compliance to Lipid-lowering Therapy in Clinical Practice', *Journal of Clinical Epidemiology*, **39**, pp. 402–409.

Scott, L.L. and Alexander J. (1998), 'Cost-effectiveness of Acyclovir Suppression to Prevent Recurrent Genital Herpes in Term Pregnancy', *American Journal of Perinatology*, **15**, pp. 57–62.

Shear, C.L., Franklin, F.A., Stinnett, S., Hurley, D.P., Bradford, R.H., Chremos, A.N., Nash, D.T. and Langendorfer, A. (1992), 'Expanded Clinical Evaluation of Lovastatin (EXCEL) Study Results. Effect of Patient Characteristics on Lovastatin-induced Changes in Plasma Concentrations of Lipids and Lipoproteins', *Circulation*, **85**, pp. 1293–303.

Simons, L.A., Levis, G. and Simons, J. (1996), 'Apparent Discontinuation Rates in Patients Prescribed Lipid-lowering Drugs', *The Medical Journal of Australia*, **164**, pp. 208–11.

Sokol, M.C., McGuigan, K.A., Verbrugge, R.R. and Epstein, R.S. (2005), 'Impact of Medication Adherence on Hospitalization Risk and Healthcare Cost', *Medical Care*, **43**(6), pp. 521–30.

Strandberg, T.E., Lehto, S., Pyorala, K., Kesaniemi, A. and Oksa, H. (1997), 'Cholesterol Lowering after Participation in the Scandinavian Simvastatin Survival Study (4S) in Finland', *European Heart Journal*, **18**, pp. 1725–27.

Taylor, J.L., Zagari, M., Murphy, K. and Freston, J.W. (1997), 'Pharmacoeconomic Comparison of Treatments for the Eradication of Helicobacter Pylori', *The Archives of Internal Medicine*, **157**, pp. 87–97.

Tonkin, A.M. (1998), 'Issues in Extrapolating from Clinical Trials to Clinical Practice and Outcomes', *Australian and New Zealand Journal of Medicine*, **28**(4), pp. 574–78.

Tu, W., Morris, A.B., Li, J., Wu, J., Young, J., Brater, D.C. and Murray, M.D. (2005), 'Association between Adherence Measurements of Metoprolol and Health Care Utilization in Older Patients with Heart Failure', *Clinical Pharmacology and Therapeutics*, **77**(3), pp. 189–201.

Urquhart, J. (1996), 'Patient Non-compliance with Drug Regimens: Measurement, Clinical Correlates, Economic Impact', *European Heart Journal*, **17**, Suppl. A, pp. 8–15.

Urquhart, J. (1997), 'The Electronic Medication Event Monitor. Lessons for Pharmacotherapy', *Clinical Pharmacokinetics*, **32**(5), pp. 345–56.

Urquhart J. (1999), 'Pharmacoeconomic Consequences of Variable Patient Compliance with Prescribed Drug Regimens', *Pharmacoeconomics*, **15**(3), pp. 217–28.

Vakil, N. and Fennerty, M.B. (1996), 'Cost-effectiveness of Treatment Regimens for the Eradication of Helicobacter Pylori in Duodenal Ulcer', *American Journal of Gastroenterology*, **91**, pp. 239–45.

Wasley, M.A., McNagny, S.E., Phillips, V.L. and Ahluwalia, J.S. (1997), 'The Cost-effectiveness of the Nicotine Transdermal Patch for Smoking Cessation', *Preventive Medicine*, **26**, pp. 264–70.

Wei, L., Wang, J., Thompson, P., Wong, S., Struthers, A.D. and MacDonald, T.M. (2002), 'Adherence to Statin Treatment and Readmission of Patients after Myocardial Infarction: A Six Year Follow up Study', *Heart*, **88**, pp. 229–30.

WOSCOPS Group (1997), 'Compliance and Adverse Event Withdrawal: Their Impact on the West of Scotland Coronary Prevention Study', *European Heart Journal*, **18**, pp. 1718–24.

Part 2
The Challenge of Compliance

Why do patients not comply? As the contributing authors explain throughout the book, the reasons are protean.

In Part 2 two, classic examples of non-compliance, cardiovascular disease and HIV infection are discussed, together with the factors influencing this decision. The perspectives gained are from Australia and France respectively, and yet the findings have worldwide resonance and relevance to anyone interested in increasing compliance in any treatment scenario. Cardiovascular disease – hypertension in particular – is usually 'silent' (without any symptoms) and yet patients are asked to engage with lifelong therapy, often taking several drugs in combination. The French have the highest consumption of medicinal products in Europe, but compliance remains a major issue; the specific, and perhaps surprising, example of non-compliance in HIV infection is used to illustrate the issues influencing the decision to comply.

CHAPTER 4

Patient Compliance in the Prevention and Treatment of Cardiovascular Disease

Professor Gregory M. Peterson and Dr Shane L. Jackson

Cardiovascular diseases (predominantly ischaemic heart disease and stroke) are amongst the leading causes of death worldwide, accounting for about one-third of global deaths or 17 million annually. That figure is expected to increase to 25 million by 2025, unless major prevention efforts can halt the rise (WHO, 2003a).

Cardiovascular disease (CVD) places a heavy burden on Australians (AIHW, 2004; Fulcher *et al.*, 2003; National Heart Foundation, 2005). It remains the major public health problem in Australia and is the leading cause of mortality and disability.

- Every ten minutes one Australian dies from CVD, accounting for 38 per cent of all deaths.
- CVD causes 22 per cent of the burden of disease in Australia.
- Compared to other diseases, CVD is the largest health cost item.
- The total financial costs of CVD are more than AU$14 billion per annum – 1.7 per cent of GDP.
- The direct health system costs of CVD were estimated at AU$7.6 billion in 2004 (11 per cent of total health spending).
- Cardiovascular disease will affect one in four Australians by 2051 (National Heart Foundation, 2005).

The proximal causes of the CVD epidemics are well known. The major risk factors –

inappropriate diet and physical inactivity (as expressed through unfavourable lipid concentrations, high body mass index and raised blood pressure), together with tobacco use – explain at least 75 per cent of new cases of CVD (Beaglehole, 2001). In the absence of these risk factors, CVD is a rare cause of death. The optimum levels of CVD risk factors are known; unfortunately, only about 5 per cent of the adult population of developed countries are at low risk with optimum risk factor levels (ibid.).

The prevention of CVD in Australia, as in many other countries, is far from optimal. For instance, according to findings in the AusDiab study in 1999–2000 (Briganti *et al.*, 2003), only 14 per cent of patients with hypertension are treated and adequately controlled, and 33 per cent are treated but not controlled. Similar figures have been reported in Canada and the United States (Joffres *et al.*, 2001; LaRosa and LaRosa, 2000).

Much of CVD can now be treated on the basis of the results of large clinical trials and can be considered 'evidence-based'. There has been an intense focus on the application of evidence-based medicine in the management of CVD, resulting in the achievement of major therapeutic advances in the treatment of conditions including hyperlipidaemia, heart failure, atrial fibrillation and hypertension. In contrast, the everyday practical use of medications (including the critical importance of patient compliance) for preventing and treating CVD has received relatively little attention. In effect, we have had a vast number of trials, conducted at huge expense, showing the potential benefits of many pharmacological agents, but only if patients take them regularly. This applies to all the cardiovascular drugs; they are possibly worthless if compliance is poor.

In viewing all aspects of patient care, it may be argued that efforts to understand and address issues of non-compliance are equally important to generating evidence of efficacy through randomized controlled trials, as patients cannot benefit from efficacious therapies unless they take them (LaRosa and LaRosa, 2000; Heidenreich, 2004; Tsuyuki and Bungard, 2001).

Two cardiovascular conditions where compliance is particularly problematic are hyperlipidaemia and hypertension – commonly occurring together and both asymptomatic conditions for which drug therapy is used to prevent long-term complications (LaRosa and LaRosa, 2000). Like hypertension and smoking, hypercholesteraemia is a chronic, painless condition that is usually perceived by the patient as having deleterious health consequences that are far in the future.

Chapman *et al.* (2005) recently examined compliance with concomitant antihypertensive and lipid-lowering drug therapy in 8406 enrollees in a US-managed care plan, who had initiated treatment with both forms of therapy within a 90-day period. Adherence was measured as the proportion of days covered in each three-month interval following initiation of concomitant therapy, with patients considered adherent if they had filled prescriptions sufficient to cover at least 80 per cent of days with both classes of medications. Less than half of patients (44.7 per cent) were adherent with both therapies three months after medication initiation, a figure that decreased to 35.8 per cent at 12 months. Adherence to antihypertensive drugs was, on average, approximately 10–15 per cent greater than with lipid-lowering medications over time. Patients were more likely to be adherent if they had initiated both treatments together, had a history of coronary heart disease or congestive heart failure, or took fewer other medications.

HYPERLIPIDAEMIA

There is extensive epidemiological evidence, from a number of large-scale studies, that relates elevation of blood total cholesterol levels to the incidence of increased coronary heart disease (Assmann *et al.*, 1998; Gotto *et al.*, 2000; National Heart Foundation and Cardiac Society, 2001; Verschuren *et al.*, 1995). In addition, many studies have now clearly demonstrated the benefits of cholesterol-lowering in patients with or without established CVD, including patients with only average cholesterol levels for Westernized societies (Gotto *et al.*, 2000; National Heart Foundation and Cardiac Society, 2001; Gould *et al.*, 1998; Bucher *et al.*, 1999; Jacobsen *et al.*, 1998).

Long-term HMG-CoA reductase inhibitor (statin) use achieves a significant reduction in mortality (24–42 per cent) for patients with coronary artery disease that is equal to or greater than that seen with other secondary prevention medications, including aspirin, beta-blockers, and angiotensin-converting enzyme (ACE) inhibitors (Smith *et al.*, 2001).

The Heart Protection Study, with over 20 500 subjects aged 40–80 years, was the largest trial of statin therapy ever conducted ('MRC/BHF', 2002; Kendall and Nuttall, 2002; Hamilton-Craig, 2002). It was a prospective double-blind randomized controlled trial investigating prolonged use (> 5 years) of simvastatin 40 mg daily and a cocktail of antioxidant vitamins (650 mg vitamin E, 250 mg vitamin C and 20 mg betacarotene daily) in patients with coronary disease, other occlusive arterial disease, or diabetes and a blood total cholesterol concentration of at least 3.5 mmol/L. Simvastatin treatment produced benefit across all patient groups regardless of age, gender or baseline cholesterol value. Results showed a 12 per cent reduction in total mortality, a 17 per cent reduction in vascular mortality, a 24 per cent reduction in CVD events, a 27 per cent reduction in all strokes and a 16 per cent reduction in non-coronary revascularizations. The antioxidant vitamin cocktail was not beneficial.

However, the translation of the clinical trial benefits of statin therapy in CVD into practice has not been easy. Under diagnosis, underuse of statin drugs and inadequate control of dyslipidaemia appear to be common worldwide (Primatesta and Poulter, 2000; Vale *et al.*, 2002a; Abookire *et al.*, 2001; Pearson *et al.*, 2000; Fonarow *et al.*, 2001; De Backer, 2002; EUROASPIRE, 2001; Yarzebski *et al.*, 2001; Van Dam *et al.*, 2002). Despite international clinical guidelines recommending lipid-lowering treatment in patients with clinically evident atherosclerotic vascular disease, study after study has documented low treatment rates in this high-risk patient population, thereby creating a clinical practice and public health dilemma (Fonarow and Watson, 2003).

Only about 30 per cent of patients with established CVD and raised serum lipids, and fewer than 10 per cent of individuals eligible for primary prevention, receive lipid-lowering therapy. Target total cholesterol concentrations are then achieved in fewer than 50 per cent of patients who do receive such treatment (Primatesta and Poulter, 2000).

Poor patient compliance to medication regimen is a major factor in the lack of success in treating hyperlipidaemia (Schedlbauer *et al.*, 2004). All of the lipid-lowering drugs must be continued indefinitely; when they are stopped, plasma cholesterol concentrations generally return to pretreatment levels (Anon, 1998). The benefits of lipid-lowering therapy will only accrue if patients comply with their medication (LaRosa and LaRosa, 2000; Schedlbauer *et al.*, 2004). The discontinuation rates with lipid-lowering therapy reported in randomized clinical trials may not reflect the rates actually observed in primary care settings (Andrade *et al.*, 1995; Avorn *et al.*, 2000). This may be a major barrier to translating the beneficial effects seen in clinical trials into everyday practice. Long-term compliance with hyperlipidaemia drugs is especially important since the major beneficial effects are seen after 12–18 months of continuous therapy (Tsuyuki and Bungard, 2001).

A study by Simons *et al.* (1996) determined that, in Australian general practice, 60 per cent of patients newly prescribed lipid-lowering drugs discontinue them within 12 months (half of these discontinuations occur within three months of initiating therapy). In a larger, Australia-wide assessment of discontinuation rates in 32 384 patients who commenced a lipid-lowering drug (statins in 92 per cent), 30 per cent had stopped taking the drug after six to seven months (Simons *et al.*, 2000). Discontinuation rates were broadly similar with all the statin drugs. The significant predictors of discontinuation were age (patients below the median age of 68 years had higher discontinuation rates) and not living in a capital city.

In a large elderly US population, only 25 per cent of patients maintained a compliance rate of at least 80 per cent with statin treatment after five years (Benner *et al.*, 2002). In a Canadian study of patients aged over 65 years, 25 per cent had discontinued statin therapy within six months of initiation (Jackevicius *et al.*, 2002). In a prospective study of hyperlipidaemic Korean patients, at six months nearly 20 per cent of the 1019 patients enrolled had discontinued treatment (Kim *et al.*, 2002).

In a study of almost 14 000 patients admitted to hospital for an acute coronary syndrome, Eagle *et al.* (2004) reported that discontinuation of drug therapy was observed at a six-month follow-up in 8 per cent of those taking aspirin on discharge, 12 per cent of those taking beta-blockers, 20 per cent of those taking ACE inhibitors, and 13 per cent of those taking statins.

Patient compliance with lipid-lowering drug therapy has even been a problem in some of the major clinical trials. Between 6 and 30 per cent of subjects enrolled in randomized controlled trials assessing the efficacy of lipid-lowering agents discontinued the study drugs (Tsuyuki and Bungard, 2001).

In the Heart Protection Study, 82 per cent of patients who received simvastatin 40 mg daily were compliant after five years, with compliance defined as at least 80 per cent of the scheduled tablets having been taken since the previous follow-up ('MRC/BHF', 2002). In the West of Scotland Coronary Prevention Study (WOSCOPS) trial (WOSCOPS, 1997; Shepherd *et al.*, 1995), almost 30 per cent of patients discontinued pravastatin over almost five years. Patients who took 75 per cent or more of their prescribed pravastatin had only one-third the risk of death from any cause compared with patients taking less than 75 per cent of the therapy (WOSCOPS, 1997; Shepherd *et al.*, 1995; Peterson *et al.*, 2003).

In a Scottish study, good compliance with statin therapy following a first myocardial infarction was associated with a reduced risk of recurrence of myocardial infarction and all-cause mortality (Wei *et al.*, 2002). There is also evidence that discontinuation of statins during acute coronary syndromes may impair vascular function independent of lipid-lowering effects. Heeschen *et al.* (2002) investigated the effects of statins on the cardiac event rate in 1616 patients of the Platelet Receptor Inhibition in Ischaemic Syndrome Management (PRISM) study who had coronary artery disease and chest pain in the previous 24 hours. Baseline clinical characteristics did not differ among 1249 patients without statin therapy, 379 patients with continued statin therapy and 86 patients with discontinued statin therapy after hospitalization. If the statin therapy was withdrawn after admission, cardiac risk increased significantly compared with patients who continued to receive statins. This was related to an increased event rate during the first week after onset of symptoms and was independent of cholesterol levels.

Given the high cost of therapy with statins (for instance, consuming almost one-quarter of the total Australian Pharmaceutical Benefits Scheme budget) and the obvious limit to society's healthcare resources, it is critical that the outcomes of lipid-lowering drug therapy are maximized (Larsen *et al.*, 2000). The reasons for poor compliance with lipid-lowering drug therapy appear to be poorly characterized and require further study (Tsuyuki and Bungard, 2001). Given the efforts of randomized controlled trials to establish the efficacy of these therapies, it is surprising that so little effort has been focused on determining compliance in clinical practice and even less in developing approaches to improve it (ibid.).

The dominant reason for non-compliance with lipid-lowering therapy in Australian patients appears to be a lack of conviction that treatment is necessary or beneficial (Simons *et al.*, 1996). Not surprisingly, patients who have experienced major cardiac events tend to be well motivated to comply with statin treatment. Larsen *et al.* (2002) reported generally good compliance with statin therapy in a Danish population, although it was noted that a high percentage of the younger patients (below 45 years of age) without drug indicators of CVD or diabetes discontinued treatment before obtaining the full benefit in terms of decreased risk of CVD morbidity and mortality. Kiortsis *et al.* (2000) also reported that younger patients were less compliant with lipid-lowering drug treatment. In their assessment of discontinuation rates in 32 384 Australian patients who commenced lipid-lowering drug therapy, Simons *et al.* (2000) reported that one of the significant predictors of discontinuation was age (patients below the median age of 68 years had higher discontinuation rates). The results of a comparative study between Funen, Denmark and Bologna, Italy indicated that compliance with lipid-lowering drug treatment appeared to be higher when used for secondary prevention (Larsen *et al.*, 2000). Together, these studies suggest that the presence of pre-existing CVD is a potent stimulus for compliance with lipid-lowering drug therapy (LaRosa and LaRosa, 2000; Schedlbauer *et al.*, 2004; Riesen *et al.*, 2004).

Although generally well tolerated, the occurrence of adverse reactions to lipid-lowering drug therapy may also pose a barrier to compliance (Kim *et al.*, 2002; Riesen *et al.*, 2004). The cost of therapy can also present a major barrier. In a study within a managed care organization in the mid-western United States, Ellis *et al.* (2004) observed a profound predictive effect of higher prescription co-payment levels on non-compliance and discontinuation of statin therapy. On average, patients receiving statins went without medication approximately 20 per cent of the time. The level of patient co-payment was an independent factor for statin discontinuation. Compared to those who had less than a US$10 co-payment, patients who paid greater than, or equal to, US$20 were more than four times more likely to discontinue their statin. In a Veterans Administration system incorporating a low patient co-payment and streamlined prescription refill procedures, persistence with the use of statins exceeded 70 per cent after 18 months of follow-up (Kopjar *et al.*, 2003). Unfortunately, the cost of medicines to patients is likely to steadily increase as governments worldwide struggle to meet the demand of growing elderly populations for expensive therapies.

HYPERTENSION

Hypertension is the most frequently managed problem in general practice in Australia, accounting for almost 9 per cent of encounters and 8 per cent of prescriptions in general practice.[6] Hypertension is a major risk factor in the development of cardiovascular disease and poses a significant public health problem. Randomized clinical trials have demonstrated that the treatment of mild-to-moderate hypertension can reduce the risk of stroke by 30 to 43 per cent and of myocardial infarction by approximately 15 per cent (WHO, 2003b; Schroeder *et al.*, 2004a, 2004b).

Despite the availability of effective treatments, the control of high blood pressure in the community is far from optimal(WHO, 2003b; Schroeder *et al.*, 2004a, 2004b; McInnes, 2004). Worldwide, less than one-quarter of hypertensive patients are adequately controlled for hypertension (Neutel and Smith, 2003). This lack of blood pressure control could be due to a wide array of possibilities including underdiagnosis and undertreatment of hypertension, and non-compliance with lifestyle modifications and medications. However, the main reason for the inadequate control of hypertension is poor compliance with the treatment regimen, both pharmacological and behavioural (for example, weight reduction, sodium intake restriction and exercise) (Thrall *et al.*, 2004).

Poor compliance with antihypertensive drug therapy in asymptomatic patients has long been recognized as a major problem (WHO, 2003b; Schroeder *et al.*, 2004a, 2004b; McInnes, 2004; Neutel and Smith, 2003; Thrall *et al.*, 2004; Krousel-Wood *et al.*, 2004; Flack *et al.*, 1996; Bloom, 1998), with 20–80 per cent of patients receiving treatment for hypertension in real-life situations considered to be 'good compliers' (WHO, 2003b). Up to half of the patients treated for hypertension drop out of care entirely within a year of diagnosis (ibid., Flack *et al.*, 1996). Consequently, approximately 75 per cent of patients with a diagnosis of hypertension do not achieve optimum blood pressure control (ibid., World Health Organization, 2003; Krousel-Wood *et al.*, 2004). Good compliance has been associated with improved blood pressure control and reduced complications of hypertension (WHO, 2003b).

PRACTICAL STRATEGIES TO PROMOTE COMPLIANCE IN CARDIOVASCULAR DISEASE

A key issue is that patients must decide to control their CVD risk factors, having understood the rationale and importance of commitment to the therapy. The healthcare provider should provide clear, direct messages about the importance of a behaviour or therapy, as well as supplying verbal and written instruction, including the rationale for treatment. Good communication skills are essential when involving the patient in decisions about treatment: active listening should be used, barriers to compliance should be anticipated and solutions discussed (LaRosa and LaRosa, 2000; National Heart Foundation, 2001; Riesen *et al.*, 2004; Miller *et al.*, 1997).

The American Heart Association expert panel on compliance recommended a multilevel approach, involving patients, healthcare providers and healthcare organizations and requiring educational and behavioural strategies. Actions that enhance compliance with prevention and treatment recommendations to reduce risk include:

1. providing clear, direct messages about importance of a behaviour or therapy
2. including patients in decisions about prevention and treatment goals and related strategies
3. incorporating behavioural strategies into counselling
4. an evidence-based practice
5. assessing patient compliance at each visit
6. developing reminder systems to ensure identification and follow-up (for example, by telephone) of patient status (Miller *et al.*, 1997).

In a study of 19 422 enrollees in a US managed care plan, who initiated treatment with a statin, Benner *et al.* (2004) concluded that early and frequent follow-up by physicians, especially with lipid testing, was associated with improved compliance to lipid-lowering therapy. However, a randomized prospective study is needed to determine whether this relationship is causal. 'Coaching' patients to adhere to both dietary advice and the drug treatment prescribed has been successful with patients with dyslipidaemia (Vale *et al.*, 2002b; Peterson *et al.*, 2004), and may be an appropriate method for reducing the treatment gap in applying evidence-based medicine to the real world (Vale *et al.*, 2002b).

Although a number of reasons for poor compliance with lipid-lowering therapy have been described, most evaluations were unsystematic, varied in content and did not allow assessment of the relative importance of the many contributing factors. In general, interventions designed to improve compliance are centred on educating patients. Until the actual mechanisms of poor compliance are known, interventions are unlikely to be focused and ultimately have a reduced likelihood of improving the situation (Tsuyuki and Bungard, 2001). Separate Cochrane reviews of strategies to improve compliance with lipid-lowering and antihypertensive drug regimens both concluded that, at this stage, no specific intervention could be recommended (Schedlbauer *et al.*, 2004; Schroeder *et al.*, 2004a). Other reviews of compliance with lipid-lowering drugs and antihypertensive therapy have drawn the same conclusion (Tsuyuki and Bungard, 2001; Peterson *et al.*, 2003; Takiya *et al.*, 2004).

The following steps have often been proposed to promote compliance with drugs used for CVD:

- Ensure that the patient understands how the proven benefits of the treatment (for example, prevention of myocardial infarction, stroke and so on) and possible ancillary benefits (for example, perhaps helping to prevent dementia or osteoporosis with statins) outweigh the inconvenience of the treatment (for example, cost or alteration of lifestyle).
- Involve the patient as a partner in all treatment decisions.
- Suggest that the patient involves their family members in their care – particularly the lifestyle changes.
- Use nurses or pharmacists to educate and monitor the patient (a number of nurse- or pharmacist-managed programmes have been very successful).
- Tailor the drug regimen to the patient's individual schedule or lifestyle and other medications.
- Prescribe once-a-day regimens whenever possible.
- Help set goals (for example, target lipid levels or blood pressure) to work towards.
- Use self-monitoring (for example, blood pressure) to promote compliance.
- Explain to the patient how they can manage any medication side-effects.
- Use calendars or diaries to remind them to take their medication.
- Use blister packs or dosette boxes to help patients remember to take their medication.
- Remind patients of due dates for prescription repeat dates.

A German study is examining the clinical and economic outcomes of a compliance-enhancing programme (including standardized contacts between the study centre and patients, mailings, telephone calls and access to a web page and hotline) with almost 8000 patients receiving rosuvastatin (Willich *et al.*, 2004).

Hypertensive patients may fail to take their medication because of the long duration of therapy, the symptomless nature of the condition, the side-effects of the medication, complicated drug regimens, lack of understanding about hypertension management and lack of motivation. Tailored combinations of strategies that include simpler dosage regimens, patient motivation and the involvement of other health professionals in a patient-centred approach are most likely to reduce the potential barriers to compliance (Schroeder *et al.*, 2004a, 2004b; Takiya *et al.*, 2004).

A Cochrane review carried out by Willich *et al.* (2004) indicated that reducing the number of daily doses appears to be effective in increasing compliance to blood pressure-lowering medication and should be tried as a first-line strategy, although there is less evidence of an effect on blood pressure reduction. Some motivational strategies and complex interventions appear promising, but more evidence is needed from randomized controlled trials.

There is now reasonable evidence that the use of new antihypertensive agents, such as the ACE inhibitors/angiotensin receptor blockers and calcium channel blockers, which are generally well-tolerated, results in improved compliance rates (McInnes, 2004; Neutel and Smith, 2003; Flack *et al.*, 1996; Bloom, 1998; Monane *et al.*, 1997; Cardinal *et al.*, 2004). Similarly, compliance may be improved by using a low-dose combination therapy of two complementary antihypertensive agents, as opposed to high-dose monotherapy with the same drugs (Neutel and Smith, 2003).

Until better insight into compliance is obtained, multifaceted measures to assist patients in following treatment with anti-hypertensives have to be adopted. The drug selected should be available, affordable, have a simple dosing regimen and, ideally, should not interfere with the patient's quality of life. Wherever feasible, patients should be taught to measure and monitor their own blood pressure and to assess their own compliance. Patients need to understand the importance of maintaining blood pressure control. Furthermore, they need to learn how to deal with missed doses, how to identify adverse events and what to do when they occur (WHO, 2003b).

CONCLUSIONS

The promotion of compliance with medications for CVD should be a major priority for governments, health professionals and the pharmaceutical industry. As noted by Elliott (2003), improving medication compliance would be a simple way of making antihypertensive drug therapies much more cost-effective. In high-risk patients, even small improvements in blood pressure control are associated with large reductions in cardiovascular risk (McInnes, 2004). Any improvement in compliance with antihypertensive and lipid-lowering medications is likely to be associated with substantial public healthcare benefits (Chapman *et al.*, 2005).

REFERENCES

Abookire, S.A., Karson, A.S., Fiskio, J., Bates, D.W. (2001), 'Use and Monitoring of 'Statin' Lipid-lowering Drugs Compared with Guidelines', *Archives of Internal Medicine*, **161**, pp. 53–58.

Andrade, S.E., Walker, A.M., Gottlieb, L.K., Hollenberg, N.K., Testa, M.A., Saperia, G.M. and Platt, R. (1995), 'Discontinuation of Antihyperlipidemic Drugs – Do Rates Reported in Clinical Trials Reflect Rates in Primary Care Settings?', *New England Journal of Medicine*, **332**, pp. 1125–31.

Anon. (1998), 'Choice of Lipid-lowering Drugs', *The Medical Letter*, **40**, pp. 117–22.

Assmann, G., Cullen, P. and Schulte, H. (1998), 'The Munster Heart Study (PROCAM). Results of Follow-up at 8 Years', *European Heart Journal*, **19**, pp. A2–11.

Australian Institute of Health and Welfare (AIHW) (2004), *Heart, Stroke and Vascular Diseases: Australian Facts 2004.* AIHW Cat. No. CVD 27, Canberra: AIHW, National Heart Foundation of Australia, National Stroke Foundation of Australia (Cardiovascular Disease Series No. 22).

Avorn, J., Monette, J., Lacour, A., Bohn, R.L., Monane, M., Mogun, H. and LeLorier, J. (1998), 'Persistence of Use of Lipid-lowering Medications: A Cross-national Study', *Journal of the American Medical Association*, **279**(18), pp. 1458–62.

Beaglehole, R. (2001), 'Global Cardiovascular Disease Prevention: Time to Get Serious', *Lancet*, **358**, pp. 661–63.

Benner, J.S., Glynn, R.J., Mogun, H., Neumann, P.J., Weinstein, M.C. and Avorn, J. (2002), 'Long-term Persistence in Use of Statin Therapy in Elderly Patients', *Journal of the American Medical Association*, **288**, pp. 455–61.

Benner, J.S., Tierce, J.C., Ballantyne, C.M., Prasad, C., Bullano, M.F., Willey, V.J. *et al.* (2004), 'Follow-up Lipid Tests and Physician Visits are Associated with Improved Adherence to Statin Therapy', *Pharmacoeconomics*, **22**, Suppl. 3, pp. 13–23.

Bloom, B.S. (1998), 'Continuation of Initial Antihypertensive Medication after 1 Year of Therapy', *Clinical Therapy*, **20**, pp. 671–81.

Briganti, E.M., Shaw, J.E., Chadban, S.J., Zimmet, P.Z., Welborn, T.A., McNeil. J.J., *et al.* (2003), 'Untreated Hypertension among Australian Adults: The 1999–2000 Australian Diabetes, Obesity and Lifestyle Study (AusDiab)', *Medical Journal of Australia*, **179**, pp. 135–39.

Bucher, H.C., Griffith, L.E. and Guyatt, G.H. (1999), 'Systematic Review on the Risk and Benefit of Different Cholesterol-lowering Interventions', *Arteriosclerosis, Thrombosis, and Vascular Biology*, **19**, pp. 187–95.

Cardinal, H., Monfared, A.A., Dorais, M., LeLorier, J. (2004), 'A Comparison between Persistence to Therapy in ALLHAT and in Everyday Clinical Practice: A Generalizability Issue', *Canadian Journal of Cardiology*, **20**, pp. 417–21.

Chapman, R.H., Benner, J.S., Petrilla, A.A., Tierce, J.C., Collins, S.R., Battleman, D.S. *et al.* (2005), 'Predictors of Adherence with Antihypertensive and Lipid-lowering Therapy', *Archives of Internal Medicine*, **165**, pp. 1147–52.

De Backer, G. (2002), 'Evidence-based Goals versus Achievement in Clinical Practice in Secondary Prevention of Coronary Heart Disease: Findings in EUROASPIRE II', *Atherosclerosis Supplements*, **2**, pp. 13–17.

Eagle, K.A., Kline-Rogers, E., Goodman, S.G., Gurfinkel, E.P., Avezum, A., Flather, M.D. *et al.* (2004), 'Adherence to Evidence-based Therapies after Discharge for Acute Coronary Syndromes: An Ongoing Prospective, Observational Study', *American Journal of Medicine*, **117**, pp. 73–81.

Elliott, W.J. (2003), 'Optimizing Medication Adherence in Older Persons with Hypertension', *International Urology and Nephrology*, **35**, pp. 557–62.

Ellis, J.J., Erickson, S.R., Stevenson, J.G., Bernstein, S.J., Stiles, R.A. and Fendrick, A.M. (2004), 'Suboptimal Statin Adherence and Discontinuation in Primary and Secondary Prevention Populations', *Journal of General Internal Medicine*, **19**, pp. 638–45.

EUROASPIRE I and II Group (2001), 'Clinical Reality of Coronary Prevention Guidelines: A Comparison of EUROASPIRE I and II in Nine Countries. EUROASPIRE I and II Group. European Action on Secondary Prevention by Intervention to Reduce Events', *Lancet*, **357**, pp. 995–1001.

Flack, J.M., Novikov, S.V. and Ferrario, C.M. (1996), 'Benefits of Adherence to Anti-hypertensive Drug Therapy', *European Heart Journal*, **17**, Suppl. A, pp. 16–20.

Fonarow, G.C. and Watson, K.E. (2003), 'Effective Strategies for Long-term Statin Use', *American Journal of Cardiology*, **92**, pp. 27i–34i.

Fonarow, G.C., French, W.J., Parsons, L.S., Sun, H. and Malmgren, J.A. (2001), 'Use of Lipid-lowering Medications at Discharge in Patients with Acute Myocardial Infarction: Data from the National Registry of Myocardial Infarction 3', *Circulation*, **103**, pp. 38–44.

Fulcher, G.R., Conner, G.W. and Amerena, J.V. (2003), 'Prevention of Cardiovascular Disease: An Evidence-based Clinical Aid', *Medical Journal of Australia*, pp. 1–14.

Gotto, A.M. Jr, Assmann, G., Carmena, R. *et al.* (2000), *The ILIB Lipid Handbook for Clinical Practice: Blood Lipids and Coronary Heart Disease* (2nd edn), New York: International Lipid Information Bureau.

Gould, A.L., Rossouw, J.E., Santanello, N.C., Heyse, J.F. and Furberg, C.D. (1998), 'Cholesterol Reduction Yields Clinical Benefit: Impact of Statin Trials', *Circulation*, **97**, pp. 946–52.

Hamilton-Craig, I. (2002), 'The Heart Protection Study: Implications for Clinical Practice', *Medical Journal of Australia*, **177**, pp. 407–408.

Heeschen, C., Hamm, C.W., Laufs, U., Bohm, M., Snapinn, S. and White, H.D. (2002), 'Withdrawal of Statins Increases Event Rates in Patients with Acute Coronary Syndromes', *Circulation*, **105**, pp. 1446–52.

Heidenreich, P.A. (2004), 'Patient Adherence: The Next Frontier in Quality Improvement', *American Journal of Medicine*, **117**, pp. 130–32.

Jackevicius, C.A., Madani, M. and Tu, J.V. (2002), 'Adherence with Statin Therapy in Elderly Patients with and without Acute Coronary Syndromes', *Journal of the American Medical Association*, **288**, pp. 462–67.

Jackson, R.T. (2001), 'Are the New Lipid Management Guidelines Good for Australia's Health? Recommendations, Possibly Resulting in the Long-term Treatment of One Million Australians, Require a Serious Cost–Benefit Analysis', *Medical Journal of Australia*, **175**, pp. 452–53.

Jacobson, T.A., Schein, J.R., Williamson, A. and Ballantyne, C.M. (1998), 'Maximizing the Cost-effectiveness of Lipid-lowering Therapy', *Archives of Internal Medicine*, **158**, pp. 1977–89.

Joffres, M.R., Ghadirian, P., Fodor, J.G., Petrasovits, A., Chockalingam, A. and Hamet, P. (1997), 'Awareness, Treatment, and Control of Hypertension in Canada', *American Journal of Hypertension*, **10**, pp. 1097–102.

Joffres, M.R., Hamet, P., MacLean, D.R., L'Italien, G.J. and Fodor, G. (2001), 'Distribution of Blood Pressure and Hypertension in Canada and the United States', *American Journal of Hypertension*, **14**, pp. 1099–105.

Kendall, M.J. and Nuttall, S.L. (2002), 'The Heart Protection Study: Statins for all those at Risk?', *Journal of Clinical Pharmacy and Therapeutics*, **27**, pp. 1–4.

Kim, Y.S., Sunwoo, S., Lee, H.R., Lee, K.M., Park, Y.W., Shin, H.C. *et al.* (2002), 'Determinants of Non-compliance with Lipid-lowering Therapy in Hyperlipidemic Patients', *Pharmacoepidemiology and Drug Safety*, **11**, pp. 593–600.

Kiortsis, D.N., Giral, P., Bruckert, E. and Turpin, G. (2000), 'Factors Associated with Low Compliance with Lipid-lowering Drugs in Hyperlipidemic Patients', *Journal of Clinical Pharmacy and Therapeutics*, **25**, pp. 445–51.

Kopjar, B., Sales, A.E., Pineros, S.L., Sun, H., Li, Y.F. and Hedeen, A.N. (2003), 'Adherence with Statin Therapy in Secondary Prevention of Coronary Heart Disease in Veterans Administration Male Population', *American Journal of Cardiology*, **92**, pp. 1106–08.

Krousel-Wood, M., Thomas, S., Muntner, P. and Morisky, D. (2004), 'Medication Adherence: A Key Factor in Achieving Blood Pressure Control and Good Clinical Outcomes in Hypertensive Patients', *Current Opinions in Cardiology*, **19**, pp. 357–62.

LaRosa, J.H. and LaRosa, J.C. (2000), 'Enhancing Drug Compliance in Lipid-lowering Treatment', *The Archives of Family Medicine*, **9**, pp. 1169–75.

Larsen, J., Vaccheri, A., Andersen, M., Montanaro, N. and Bergman, U. (2000), 'Lack of Adherence to Lipid-lowering Drug Treatment. A Comparison of Utilization Patterns in Defined Populations in Funen, Denmark and Bologna, Italy', *British Journal of Clinical Pharmacology*, **49**, pp. 463–71.

Larsen, J., Andersen, M., Kragstrup, J. and Gram, L.F. (2002), 'High Persistence of Statin Use in a Danish Population: Compliance Study 1993–1998', *British Journal of Clinical Pharmacology*, **53**, pp. 375–78.

McInnes, G.T. (2004), 'How Important is Optimal Blood Pressure Control?', *Clinical Therapy*, **26**, Suppl. A, pp. A3–11.

Miller, N.H., Hill, M., Kottke, T. and Ockene, I.S. (1997), 'The Multilevel Compliance Challenge: Recommendations for a Call to Action: A Statement for Healthcare Professionals', *Circulation*, **95**, pp. 1085–90.

Monane, M., Bohn, R.L., Gurwitz, J.H., Glynn, R.J., Levin, R. and Avorn, J. (1997), 'The Effects of Initial Drug Choice and Comorbidity on Antihypertensive Therapy Compliance: Results from a Population-based Study in the Elderly', *American Journal of Hypertension*, **10**, pp. 697–704.

'MRC/BHF Heart Protection Study of Cholesterol Lowering with Simvastatin in 20,536 High-risk Individuals: A Randomised Placebo-controlled Trial', *Lancet*, **360**, pp. 7–22.

Neutel, J.M. and Smith, D.H. (2003), 'Improving Patient Compliance: A Major Goal in the Management of Hypertension', *Journal of Clinical Hypertension*, **5**, pp. 127–32.

National Heart Foundation of Australia (2005), *The Shifting Burden of Cardiovascular Disease*, Report prepared by Access Economics.

National Heart Foundation of Australia and the Cardiac Society of Australia and New Zealand (2001), 'Lipid Management Guidelines – 2001', *Medical Journal of Australia*, **175** (Suppl.), pp. S57–S88.

Pearson, T.A., Laurora, I., Chu, H. and Kafonek, S. (2000), 'The Lipid Treatment Assessment Project (L-TAP): A Multicenter Survey to Evaluate the Percentages of Dyslipidemic Patients Receiving Lipid-lowering Therapy and Achieving Low-density Lipoprotein Cholesterol Goals', *Archives of Internal Medicine*, **160**, pp. 459–67.

Peterson, A.M., Takiya, L. and Finley, R. (2003), 'Meta-analysis of Interventions to Improve Drug Adherence in Patients with Hyperlipidemia', *Pharmacotherapy*, **23**, pp. 80–87.

Peterson, G.M., Fitzmaurice, K.D., Naunton, M., Vial, J.H., Stewart, K. and Krum, H. (2004), 'Impact of Pharmacist-conducted Home Visits on the Outcomes of Lipid-lowering Drug Therapy', *Journal of Clinical Pharmacy and Therapeutics*, **29**, pp. 23–30.

Primatesta, P. and Poulter, N.R. (2000), 'Lipid Concentrations and the Use of Lipid Lowering Drugs: Evidence from a National Cross Sectional Survey', *British Medical Journal*, **321**, pp. 1322–25.

Riesen, W.F., Darioli, R. and Noll, G. (2004), 'Lipid-lowering Therapy: Strategies for Improving Compliance', *Current Medical Research and Opinion*, **20**, pp. 165–73.

Schedlbauer, A., Schroeder, K., Peters, T.J. and Fahey, T. (2004), 'Interventions to Improve Adherence to Lipid Lowering Medication', *Cochrane Database System Review*, CD004371.

Schroeder, K., Fahey, T. and Ebrahim, S. (2004a), 'How Can We Improve Adherence to Blood Pressure-lowering Medication in Ambulatory Care? Systematic Review of Randomized Controlled Trials', *Archives of Internal Medicine*, **164**, pp. 722–32.

Schroeder, K., Fahey, T. and Ebrahim, S. (2004b), 'Interventions for Improving Adherence to Treatment in Patients with High Blood Pressure in Ambulatory Settings', *Cochrane Database System Review*, CD004804.

Shepherd, J., Cobbe, S.M., Ford, I., Isles, C.G., Lorimer, A.R., MacFarlane, P.W. *et al.* (1995), 'Prevention of Coronary Heart Disease with Pravastatin in Men with Hypercholesterolemia', *New England Journal of Medicine*, **333**, pp. 1301–07.

Simons, L.A., Levis, G. and Simons, J. (1996), 'Apparent Discontinuation Rates in Patients Prescribed Lipid-lowering Drugs', *The Medical Journal of Australia*, **164**, pp. 208–11.

Simons L.A., Simons, J., McManus, P. and Dudley, J. (2000), 'Discontinuation Rates for Use of Statins are High', *British Medical Journal*, **321**, p. 1084.

Smith, S.C. Jr, Blair, S.N., Bonow, R.O., Brass, L.M., Cerqueira, M.D., Dracup, K. *et al.* (2001), 'AHA/ACC Scientific Statement: AHA/ACC Guidelines for Preventing Heart Attack and Death in Patients with Atherosclerotic Cardiovascular Disease: 2001 Update: A Statement for Healthcare Professionals from the American Heart Association and the American College of Cardiology', *Circulation*, **104**, pp. 1577–79.

Takiya, L.N., Peterson, A.M. and Finley, R.S. (2004), 'Meta-analysis of Interventions for Medication Adherence to Antihypertensives', *The Annals of Pharmacotherapy*, **38**, pp. 1617–24.

Thrall, G., Lip, G.Y. and Lane, D. (2004), 'Compliance with Pharmacological Therapy in Hypertension: Can We Do Better, and How?', *Journal of Human Hypertension*, **18**, pp. 595–97.

Tsuyuki, R.T. and Bungard, T.J. (2001), 'Poor Adherence with Hypolipidemic Drugs: A Lost Opportunity', *Pharmacotherapy*, **21**, pp. 576–82.

Vale, M.J., Jelinek, M.V., Best, J.D. for the COACH Study Group (2002a), 'How Many Patients with Coronary Heart Disease are not Achieving their Risk-factor Targets? Experience in Victoria 1996–1998 versus 1999–2000', *Medical Journal of Australia*, **176**, pp. 211–15.

Vale, M.J., Jelinek, M.V., Best, J.D. and Santamaria, J.D. (2002b), 'Coaching Patients with Coronary Heart Disease to Achieve the Target Cholesterol: A Method to Bridge the Gap between Evidence-based Medicine and the "Real World" – Randomized Controlled Trial', *Journal of Clinical Epidemiology*, **55**, pp. 245–52.

Van Dam, M., Van Wissen, S. and Kastelein, J.J. (2002), 'Declaring War on Undertreatment: Rationale for an Aggressive Approach to Lowering Cholesterol', *Journal of Cardiovascular Risk*, **9**, pp. 89–95.

Verschuren, W.M., Jacobs, D.R., Bloemberg, B.P., Kromhout, D., Menotti, A., Aravanis, C. *et al.* (1995), 'Serum Total Cholesterol and Long-term Coronary Heart Disease Mortality in Different Cultures: Twenty-five-year Follow-up of the Seven Countries Study', *Journal of the American Medical Association*, **274**, 131–36.

Wei, L., Wang, J., Thompson, P., Wong, S., Struthers, A.D. and MacDonald, T.M. (2002), 'Adherence to Statin Treatment and Readmission of Patients after Myocardial Infarction: A Six Year Follow up Study', *Heart*, **88**, pp. 229–30.

WHO (2003a), 'Neglected Global Epidemics: Three Growing Threats', in *The World Health Report 2003 – Shaping the Future*, Geneva: World Health Organization, pp. 83–102.

WHO (2003b), 'Adherence to Long-term Therapies: Evidence for Action, July at: http://www.who.int/chronic_conditions/adherencereport/en/index.html (accessed July 2005).

Willich, S.N., Muller-Nordhorn, J., Sonntag, F., Voller, H., Meyer-Sabellek, W., Wegscheider, K., *et al.* (2004), 'Economic Evaluation of a Compliance-enhancing Intervention in Patients with Hypercholesterolemia: Design and baseline results of the Open Label Primary Care Study: Rosuvastatin Based Compliance Initiatives To Achievements of LDL Goals (ORBITAL) Study', *American Heart Journal*, **148**, pp. 1060–67.

WOSCOPS Group (1997), 'Compliance and Adverse Event Withdrawal: Their Impact on the West of Scotland Coronary Prevention Study', *European Heart Journal*, **18**, pp. 1718–24.

Yarzebski, J., Spencer, F., Goldberg, R.J., Lessard, D. and Gore, J.M. (2001), 'Temporal Trends (1986–1997) in Cholesterol Level Assessment and Management Practices in Patients with Acute Myocardial Infarction – A Population-based Perspective', *Archives of Internal Medicine*, **161**, pp. 1521–28.

CHAPTER 5

Patient Compliance: A French Perspective

Catherine Narayan-Dubois

One of the primary aims of the French healthcare system is to ensure that its citizens remain in good health. In France, people are justifiably proud that the French healthcare system was concluded to be the best in the world in the World Health Organization's 2000 ranking of healthcare systems (Izmirlieva, 2004). However, this high-quality service has come at a price. Around 75 per cent of total health spending is publicly funded, and citizens have fewer out-of-pocket expenses for medical treatment and prescriptions than citizens of other major industrialized countries (ibid.). To understand how medicines are prescribed in France, and the factors important in patient compliance, it is necessary to briefly examine the background to healthcare in the country. As with other countries, the attitudes of patients, prescribers and pharmaceutical companies combined with the nature of the pricing system all play a role in the use of medicines.

HEALTHCARE

One of the features of pharmaceuticals is that governments are often directly or indirectly involved in paying the consumer's bills. This means that, in countries where the government burden is high, there is a strong incentive for them to try to reduce the per capita cost. France remains one of the highest-spending nations on pharmaceuticals; consequently, successive governments have pursued cost containment policies as a means of driving down this spend, but patients have opposed any measures that would result in them paying higher prices for healthcare. In France, as patients have fairly affordable access to medicines they are less price-conscious than their counterparts in other countries and this is reflected in the population's high use of medicines. A recent survey by the Organization for Economic Co-operation and Development (OECD) revealed that pharmaceuticals accounted for more than 10 per cent of total health spending in most countries, but that in France they accounted for over 20 per cent of this sum (OECD, 2003). A combination of low prices and a high level of government reimbursement give patients and physicians little incentive to cut consumption (Kermani, 2004).

At the time of writing, there are a total of 4056 medicinal products on the French market, and the quantity of medicinal products sold per inhabitant in France by pharmaceutical companies is the highest in Europe. Furthermore, according to the French pharmaceutical industry body, LEEF (Les entreprises du médicament), since 1995 France has been the leading drug-producing nation within the European Union and remains the third largest producer of pharmaceuticals worldwide (Pharmaceutiques, 2002).

The main prescribers of medicines in France are essentially the physicians: general practitioners or specialists and, to some extent, dentists and midwives. The details of the medicines that dentists and midwives are permitted to prescribe are listed in the Public Health Code, which defines the rules regarding healthcare. In France there are currently 196 000 physicians, of whom 99 250 are specialists, providing approximately 331 physicians for every 100 000 inhabitants. This figure is considerably higher than the 175 physicians for every 100 000 inhabitants in the UK and the 464 physicians per 100 000 in Germany. In addition, the French ratio has more than doubled over the last 30 years. For example, in 1970 there were only 130 physicians for every 100 000 patients in France (Pharmaceutiques, 2002).

The majority of pharmacies in France are privately operated and owned by one or several pharmacists. The Public Health Code defines the number of permitted pharmacies per inhabitants. Recent estimates suggest that there is one pharmacy for every 3000 inhabitants in France. Other types of pharmacies in France include those that are hospital-based or are part of a private clinic. These pharmacies are only allowed to dispense the medication prescribed for their in-patients.

Medicinal products on the French market are generally classified into prescription-only medicines and over-the-counter (OTC) medicines (that is, medicines which may be bought by consumers from a pharmacy without a prescription). Irrespective of the class that a medicine belongs to, only a pharmacist is allowed to dispense such products. There are specific examples of medicines with restricted dispensing from a hospital pharmacy only – for example, certain classes of antibiotics. In each class, medicinal products that are made available are categorized as branded products or generics.

The French social security system offers partial reimbursement of the physicians' fees. Depending on the agreement that each physician, general practitioner or specialist has signed with the security social organization, the Caisse Nationale d'Assurance Maladie (CNAM), the patient will be reimbursed for varying amounts. The majority of physicians are designated 'conventionné', whereby they agree the fees proposed by the CNAM. Each time patients visit a physician belonging to this group, they will be reimbursed for 70 per cent of the price of the visit, and this level of reimbursement is the same for all physicians of this group.

A second group of physicians are known as *conventionnés honoraires libres*. To a certain extent, the fees requested by these physicians are higher than the fees proposed by the CNAM. However, patients will be reimbursed for the same amount of money as if they had consulted a *conventionné* physician. The last group of physicians, who represent a very small percentage of those qualified to practise in France, have refused to sign either agreement. In these cases, visit fees are very high and the patient is not reimbursed.

As well as physician fees, all prescription-only medication expenses are reimbursed to the patient through the CNAM system. Three levels of reimbursement of prescription-only medications have been defined according to criteria known as the *service médical rendu*. On a regular basis a commission of experts evaluates each product and then determines its reimbursement rate on the basis of its efficacy in the claimed indication compared to the existing therapeutic alternatives. The reimbursement rate for a particular product may change during its life cycle.

The CNAM reimburses the full price of all products used to treat 'very serious disorders', such as HIV infection. The next class of products are those designated to treat or cure a 'serious disorder' such as hypertension or asthma, which are reimbursed at the rate of 65 per cent. For 'non-serious disorders', the CNAM reimburses 35 per cent of the prices of products. In all these cases, the patient pays the remaining amount. This cost will be met by the patients personally if they cannot afford individual private medical insurance.

France established a comprehensive system of social security in 1946, after the Second World War. Social security is a right of citizenship in France: the constitution explicitly guarantees a certain minimum standard of living and healthcare for all French citizens. France spends about 29 per cent of its annual gross domestic product (GDP) on social security, significantly more than is spent in the UK or the United States. Universal, compulsory social insurance reimburses much of the cost of healthcare (Embassy of France, 2001). The social security system is financed largely from payroll and savings taxes, with a smaller percentage contributed from the national government's general budget.

Are all patients entitled to be reimbursed?

Nearly all of the French population is covered by the social security system. The patients pay the outstanding portion of the physician's fees or prescribed medication expenses when they have no personal insurance, as is the case for about 15 per cent of the population. According to a survey, 61 per cent of the pharmacy expenses per patient are reimbursed by the CNAM, 19 per cent by private insurance, and the patient pays the remaining 20 per cent (Embassy of France, 2001). Patients choose their general practitioners as well as specialists. Furthermore, they can go to any pharmacy of their choice to purchase their medicines.

In many cases, the patient has to pay the physician upfront and the CNAM and/or personal insurance then directly reimburses the patient upon presentation of a certificate called the '*Feuille de soin*' issued by the physician. However, the system is different for pharmacies. In many cases, the patient provides the pharmacist with proof of registration with the CNAM and a personal insurance company. The patient then pays nothing directly as the pharmacist sends the cost of the medication entitled to be reimbursed to both these bodies which will then reimburse the pharmacist within a three-month timeframe. This system is called *tiers-payant*. A patient can be registered with different pharmacies.

COMPLIANCE

In France the terminology for compliance is associated with 'observance' and derives its meaning and connotations from its historical interpretation in the context of religion during the Middle Ages. In the French sense, compliance can be taken to mean that the patient should follow the prescription or advice provided by the physician 'religiously'. In the modern-day French context, compliance denotes the extent to which medications are taken in the dosage and frequency agreed between the prescriber and patient. Compliance encompasses prescribed medicinal products as well as verbal information provided by the physician. A lack of such compliance, in effect undercompliance, is more common than overcompliance.

Undercompliance is considered to pertain to situations where the patient deliberately does not take medication, where patients consciously omit their medication, or inadvertently do not take their medication (or where the patient cannot take their medication), and where patients have difficulties assessing or remembering to take their medication. Non-compliance can put the patient in danger. Indeed, undercompliance reduces the efficacy of the treatment. In diseases such as depression, undercompliance increases the risk of suicide, which is tackled by the intake of the drug. In contrast, overcompliance, in terms of (accidental) overdose or polypharmacy, provokes side-effects.

In France, as elsewhere, it has been noted that patients demonstrate non-compliance with both prescription-only and OTC medicines. Whereas overcompliance is generally observed with OTC products, patients are mainly undercompliant with their prescribed medicines.

A survey conducted on prescription-only products revealed that only half of French patients (53 per cent) are compliant with their prescription, with the remainder failing to adhere to the duration of treatment or the dosage prescribed. Of this group, 26 per cent declared that they acted in this manner 'sometimes' (19 per cent) or 'often' (7 per cent) (Maillard, 2003).

When non-compliance has been studied in greater depth for long-term disorders, it has been found, perhaps surprisingly, to be an issue relevant to all therapeutic classes and all types of disease. For example, non-compliance has been noted with medicines for the treatment of metabolic diseases such as hypercholesterolaemia or type II diabetes, and in long-term conditions such as hypertension or asthma. Furthermore, patients suffering from serious infections do not take their prescribed medicines as directed. Indeed, 57 per cent of patients suffering from HIV infection are not considered to be compliant (Actions

Traitements, 2004). In these cases, non-compliance was noticed only when patients were hospitalized after suffering from the serious effects of their illness. In the past there was little evaluation of such patients, but as the importance of non-compliance has become recognized, systems to measure how patients comply with their prescribed anti-HIV treatment have been established.

How can compliance be measured?

In France, as is the case in other countries, there is no universally accepted measurement for the state of patient compliance. A standard approach has been to assess the manner in which a patient complies with the treatment prescribed through the use of a questionnaire. However, the weakness of this approach is that patients tends only to remember the manner in which they have taken their medicine over the last two days or so and earlier information cannot be considered reliable. To address this issue, electronic approaches, such as the use of pill-counting dispensers can be used, and these can be backed up by a pharmacist's own assessment of the amount of remaining medication.

What does a medicinal product actually mean to the patient?

Various reports in France have shown that the way in which a patient thinks about a medicinal product can depend on age as well as on health status (Maillard, 2003; Actions Traitements, 2004; Bonet and Maillard, 2003; Ipsos/Assurance Maladie, 2002). For example, amongst adults (20–40 years of age) there can be a surprising distrust of the medicine prescribed. Because the medicinal product is a chemical product, it may be considered potentially dangerous and the patient may be rather unwilling to take it compared to, for example, a herbal product, which the patient considers to be 'safe'. These respondents express fears concerning side-effects and have concerns about the risk of becoming too dependent on a product.

Respondents in the 50+ age group tend to be more critical. Even though the majority express a degree of trust in the drug, many remain fearful of side-effects inherent in the product itself or caused by polypharmacy, and of the risk of dependency. Many of those who express trust in a product do so because their fear of the disease being treated is greater than their fear of the possible adverse effects of the drug they are taking to cure it.

Patients in the 60+ age group have a different opinion concerning medical products and this is no doubt due to the fact that the majority are accustomed to taking medicines. Some among this category of patients often consider the product prescribed to have potential dangers, but they continue to take their medicine as it is seen as a means to maintaining a high quality of life, enabling them to carry out normal everyday tasks. They tend to accept the possibility of side-effects from the medicine, believing that this is an unavoidable risk associated with using the medicine and they evaluate this risk in the general context of how they wish to live their life avoiding ill-health and possible dependency upon others.

Another reason for the different opinions of this category of patients regarding medicines is that they are old enough to have witnessed a tremendous change in the healthcare situation in France and appreciate the benefits that modern medicines can bring to their daily lives. For example, in the 1930s very few people could afford to go to a physician, and a drug would have only been prescribed in extreme circumstances. During this time in France, deaths from conditions such as asthma, bronchitis and tetanus were commonplace. Thus, from the perspective of these patients, when free access to medicinal products was introduced after the Second World War through the implementation of Social Security, medicines became an essential part of their everyday lives.

This category of patient is thus able to appreciate what a drug has brought to society and has personal recollections of having seen major diseases and the personal misery of their effects eradicated. Consequently, these patients trust the prescriber as well as the products they prescribe. In fact, in contrast to adults in the 20–40 year age group, they express a distrust of all herbal medicinal products or traditional medicines.

Interestingly, children also trust both the physician and the drug. The drug prescribed by the physician is seen as a means to treat or cure a disease; in their eyes that drug is, for example, the 'super hero who fights the bacteria and wins'! Consequently, drugs such as painkillers or hypnotics are not seen as real medicines. It has been noted that children are aware of the risks of overcompliance and are aware that overdose or polypharmacy can lead to death.

Compliance in a dynamic context

A lack of compliance is essentially due to combined factors as described above. It should be considered as a dynamic phenomenon which changes in time. The same patient will not be compliant in the same way over time even if there is no change in extrinsic factors. Some of the observations below are based on my own experience of working as a pharmacist in France.

Patients take their medicines when the disease they suffer from is accompanied by symptoms which make them feel conscious of the disease. What tends to occur is that patients remain compliant with the medication prescribed while the symptoms prevent them from leading a normal life. This is the case when diseases are associated with pain. In my own experience there tends to be good compliance with painkillers.

In contrast, I have observed that patients suffering from asymptomatic, but potentially serious, metabolic diseases such as hypercholesterolaemia or type II diabetes are less compliant with their medicines. As the only sign of the disorder they suffer from is an abnormal haematology or biochemistry, it generally tends to have little direct meaning for the patient. In the case of asthma, the majority of patients take medicines when they suffer from an asthma attack, as this is when they become conscious of the disorder having an immediate impact on their daily life.

In addition to being aware of the disorder they suffer from, the patients must accept their condition in order to be compliant. This lack of acceptance is a very common phenomenon in conditions such as HIV infection (Bême and Guénot, 2002), epilepsy or mental disorders such as depression or schizophrenia. The fact that such diseases are still considered to be taboo by society in general certainly does not help the situation. The same fear remains for sexually transmitted diseases, even though treatment options exist.

If the symptoms influence the way in which the patient complies with the prescription, then the complexity and the length of the treatment are also of key importance. This is known to be particularly the case for a long-term condition such as HIV infection (ibid.). In HIV infection, a compliance rate of at least 95 per cent is required to get the best result and to reduce the risk of viral resistance to the medication. The majority of anti-HIV medication has to be taken two or three times per day within a regular timeframe in order to reach a high blood concentration and it must be taken over many years. Special warnings apply to the intake of such medicines (intake with food or water). Such regimens require complicated pill schedules that could confound even the most diligent and organized individuals. The difficulty with compliance is increased when the patient feels it necessary to hide the medication from family or colleagues.

A survey conducted in 668 seropositive women in France in 2002 revealed new key criteria that had an impact in preventing the patient from being compliant (ibid.). Among common factors that will be examined later in this chapter, socioeconomic factors were of key importance. This survey showed that only 56 per cent of women were compliant whereas the corresponding figure for men was 69 per cent. The reason was that the majority of women surveyed did not have a stable home and had a very low income. Indeed, for a patient who lives in an economically deprived area and doesn't have a fridge, keeping a medication refrigerated was quite impossible. Also, one-third of those surveyed were suffering from depression, leading to excessive intake of alcohol or narcotics.

The medicine itself

The nature of the drug itself and its effects can have a strong bearing on the degree of patient compliance. Patients expect a drug to treat a disease or symptoms, not to provide discomfort or further symptoms. The concept of risk–benefit assessment is largely unfamiliar to the population and, even in cases where patients are aware of the potential risk and seem to accept it, their attitude will change when they suffer from a side-effect. Few patients will call the physician or the pharmacist for advice. Usually, they change the dosage or simply stop taking the medicine.

The dosage form also plays an active role in the way in which the patient complies with the prescription. Patients do not consider different forms of a medicinal drug to have equal importance. Indeed, many patients of all age groups tend to classify a medicine according to the dosage form, not the active ingredient. In this scale of value the most respected form according to the average French patient is the injectable medicine. The patient will comply with an injection formulation religiously as the medicine is perceived to be a 'real' medicine and that the disease they suffer from is serious. According to the patient's perceived view, the injectable form is a medicine that 'deserves' to be taken according to the strict requirements of the prescriber. Moreover, a nurse may administer the injection as the patient is often in a hospital setting and this confers even greater importance upon the product.

After the injectable form, oral dosage forms are held in high regard by French patients. These include capsules, hard capsules and tablets, which are usually referred to by patients as a *cachet*. As these forms are swallowed, patients tend to associate them with serious diseases or disorders such as metabolic disease, hypertension and cardiac diseases.

French patients associate syrups with very mild infections, which result in symptoms such as a cough. In addition to suppositories, they are the formulation often given to children. Both of them are kept in the house with food; suppositories are often kept in the fridge and syrups are generally stored in the kitchen cupboard with the sweets. Topical forms of medicines such as ointments, creams or gels are seen as cosmetic and are usually kept in the bathroom with items such as moisturizers and cosmetic products. Consequently, the disorders that these products are used to treat are not perceived as serious conditions.

Apart from the way in which the patient thinks about the medicines, the formulation prescribed should be evaluated for its appropriateness for particular patients in terms of their lifestyle, age or health condition. For example, many prescriptions for elderly people involve a dosage form such as drops, yet their use requires a certain level of physical ability and coordination, which a patient of this age may no longer possess. The same problem can be encountered with scored tablets, which the patient is unable to break into two pieces. As a consequence, the patient may take the whole tablet rather than the half intended.

Non-compliance is also due to factors inherent in the patient. Amongst various other factors, the social group that the patient belongs to heavily influences his or her interaction with the physician and any medicines prescribed. Patients with a good level of education and adequate financial means will be more compliant than their poorer counterparts in the way in which they buy medicines that are not reimbursed by the health system. At the same time, the more affluent patients tend to have better medical knowledge, which has been obtained from television, the Internet or magazines. However, it is well known that patients who turn to these information sources are also more demanding in the type of treatment and medical care that they seek.

Patients still respect their prescriber, but they are willing to challenge their physician in a manner that would not have occurred a decade ago. The doctor–patient relationship has changed, and the physician is seen as a human being who can provide the wrong diagnosis or prescription. Many general practitioners believe that patients are now more demanding than ever before. One interesting observation is that the greater the degree of education these respondents possess, the less trust they seem to place in their physicians. As they often possess professional qualifications themselves they may be under the impression that they have the ability to critically evaluate the physician's decision. As a result, they may have sufficient self-confidence to challenge the physician's judgement.

Nowadays, the average French patient has effectively become a 'consumer' and the French physician has become a 'product'. If patients are not happy with the diagnosis provided or the medicines prescribed, they simply take their custom to another physician. In France, this increasingly common phenomenon is known as *tourisme medical* (medical tourism). It is not uncommon to find French patients who will openly talk about seeing a second physician because they either distrust the efficacy of the original prescription they were given or because the medicines prescribed were not those that they expected. These patients will even criticize their original physician's decisions in front of another physician.

Religious beliefs may also have a bearing on patients' attitudes towards the prescription (Loriol, 2002). According to one survey that was conducted with 180 French patients and concerned their religious background, Catholic and Muslim respondents expressed the greatest degree of trust in their physician and, to a lower degree, in their pharmacist. Respondents who identified themselves as Jewish appeared to have a more critical attitude and seemed prepared to argue with the physician if necessary, whereas Protestants showed a more independent attitude. Indeed, it was not unusual to find that some of these patients copied the prescription and destroyed the original, as if they wished to portray themselves as the original writer of that prescription! Some patients in this survey indicated that they would not take psychotropic drugs. Catholic respondents indicated that they would not take such medicines because of a fear of putting on weight, whereas Protestant respondents expressed concerns about of becoming dependent on the product. Loss of memory was the main argument raised by the Jewish respondents, whereas Muslim respondents expressed their reservations about loss of control and risk of madness. Although this was a small survey, it highlights how a variety of factors in patients' backgrounds, such as religious beliefs, may have an influence over their attitudes to compliance and their reasons for non-compliance.

Medical tourism

In a situation where patients tend to practise medical tourism, physicians now try to maintain a good relationship with them because they have become, in effect, clients. The only physicians whom French patients appear to trust are professors. The aura surrounding the status and the white coat still has an impact on most patients, who follow the prescription and advice provided by the professor with almost religious zeal.

The concept of medical tourism applies to the pharmacist as well. Indeed, whereas the physician is still seen as an educated professional (on account of the length of study, the difficulties in gaining access to the profession and the fact that medicine is a vocation all parents still desire their children to take up), a pharmacist is perceived differently. Indeed, the pharmacist is generally seen more as a vendor than the expert on the drug being dispensed. Their qualifications are often not recognized and their monopoly on dispensing medications is often criticized. This is a pity as a better relationship between the patient and the pharmacist, as well as between the patient and physician would definitely improve compliance.

The only opportunity for a pharmacist to note a lack of compliance is when the patient comes to the pharmacy to renew their prescription – that is, every month according to the Code of Public Health. However, even if lack of compliance can be noticed through the amount of remaining drug in the packaging, the pharmacist cannot check compliance in terms of the time of intake. In many cases, the advice provided by the pharmacist consists of writing the daily dosage on the packaging, which is not designed for that purpose.

How can this lack of compliance be tackled?

In many long-term conditions, such as HIV infection or hypertension, reducing the quantity of medication may be difficult, as each associated condition has to be treated.

With the elderly it is important to help the patient remember to take their medicine or ensure that they are able to gain access to it, as these factors can lead to non-compliance. Pharmaceutical companies should ensure that the medication is available in appropriate packaging, which is easily opened by the older patient – that is, avoiding childproof containers or blister packs which require strength to open them.

As well as the packaging, the pharmaceutical industry should make available appropriate formulations for the category of patients it aims to treat. For example, drops are definitely not suitable for elderly, whose visual acuity is very low. Similarly, syrups are the most appropriate form for children. Formulating for compliance is discussed in detail by Dr Kusai in Chapter 7 of this book.

As patients refer to, and recognize, the formulation or the packaging more than the international non-proprietary names (INNs), any change in the size, shape or colour of the formulation or the packaging may affect compliance.

The same issue is encountered when the physician or pharmacist proposes a switch from proprietary to generic medication – the tablet or capsule has to be the same. If it is not, patients may convince themselves that the new tablets are not the same and could be associated with side-effects, even though the generic form would not produce these effects.

Appropriate dosage strengths must also be made available to the patient. For example, lower dosages are required for the elderly, particularly when initiating treatment. Lower dosages of oral formulated drugs are often not marketed, which leads to the need to break higher-strength or scored tablets. This should be avoided since they can be difficult for elderly patients to break, and the resulting dose used in practice by these individuals may be inaccurate.

Simply forgetting to take a medicine can be a common reason for non-compliance and there can be a variety of factors that lead to this situation. In the case of polypharmacy dispensing devices, which divide weekly amounts of drugs into separate daily doses so that they can be taken at the correct time, are useful and have already proved their efficacy in improving compliance amongst the elderly (Garcia-Ficheux, 2005). New systems such as alarms and Short Message Services have already proved to be of great help in helping asthmatic adolescents to remember to use their inhalers. However, such devices are costly and will not be financed by the Social Security system, particularly as the main concerns of the current French government are to reduce the costs of healthcare.

Information overload

Information on diseases or drugs gathered by the patient is now available through a range of diverse sources, and these have increased dramatically over the last ten years. There are numerous magazines, websites and CD-ROMs listing all the medications marketed in France, with their indications, warnings, side-effects and dosage. A version of the Vidal, considered to be the equivalent to the British Medicines Compendium or American Physicians Desk Reference (PDR), which is the prescription reference book used by physicians, is available to the French patient. Yet this wide availability of medical information does not mean that patients are receiving the correct information, nor does it mean that the conclusions they reach about their treatments and medicines are correct. In fact, much of this information is not sufficiently technical to be used for practical medical purposes and can lead to patients becoming confused about the disease they are suffering from or the medicine they are taking. Moreover, it must be remembered that each patient will tend to understand the information in relation to his or her educational and socioeconomic background. In many cases, patients visit the physician or the pharmacist with erroneous information concerning the condition that they suffer from. For example, from my own experiences, it is not unusual to hear of patients refusing antibiotics because they believe that such medicines will make them feel tired.

It is not only the media that bombard patients with potential medical information. Further information on medicines is provided by the French health authorities. In many cases they run their own public advertising campaigns, focusing, for example, on antibiotics and the consequence of excessive consumption of such medicines. These campaigns are aimed at encouraging patients to take a greater interest in their own healthcare, whilst also aiming to reduce costs borne by the government. Although such campaigns increase patient awareness of the consequences of the excessive use of medicines, they can also have a negative impact on compliance as they act to reinforce the patient's suspicions that the medicines they take may have unwanted side-effects. As a result, these patients may decide not to adhere to their recommended treatment, and their relationship with the physician will be affected. They may even consider switching to another physician who they feel supports their negative view of a particular medical product.

Information provided on the diseases or drug should involve both the physician and pharmacist or should be supplied directly by them. Information from other sources must be treated with caution, as its relevance to the healthcare status of the patient is unknown until an expert is able to assess its content.

OUTLOOK AND CONCLUSION

Currently a variety of measures are being developed to try to reduce medical tourism in France, but it is unclear whether they will have the desired effect in terms of patient compliance. Patient compliance remains a multifaceted problem with no easy solution.

Pharmaceutical companies are developing ever more innovative and sophisticated forms of their products, but patients need to understand the nature of these medicines for them to be effective. It will be important for more responsibility, as well as more financial incentives, to be given to French physicians and pharmacists so that they feel comfortable in spending extra time with their patients to ensure that compliance issues are addressed. This will allow patients to better understand how the medicine prescribed relates to their condition and will encourage them to take it in the required manner.

REFERENCES

Actions Traitements (2004), 'Vous avez dit observance?', 1 January at: http://www.actions-traitements.org/article.php3?id_article=445.

Bême, D. and Guéniot, C. (2002), 'La précarité handicape l'observance' at: http://www.doctissimo.fr.

Bonet, P. and Maillard C. (2003), 'Les médicaments et les Français: quelles solutions pour un meilleur usage?', *Concours Médical*, **125**(19), pp. 1039–42.

Embassy of France in the United States (2001), 'French Society', 26 February at: http://www.ambafrance-us.org/atoz/social.asp.

Garcia-Ficheux, F. (2005), 'N'oubliez plus vos médicaments' at: http://www.doctissimo.fr/html/medicaments/articles/sa_6362_medicaments_oubli_astuces.htm.

Ipsos/Assurance Maladie (2002), 'Regards croisés médecins-patients sur la relation aux antibiotiques', *Synthèse*, June at: http://www.cpam-dordogne.fr/PDF/RCMPSLRAA.pdf.

Izmirlieva M. (2004), 'French Healthcare Reform: Economic Realities Prompt Departure from "World's Best Healthcare System"', PricewaterhouseCoopers at:. http://www.pwcglobal.com/Extweb/NewCoAtWork.nsf/docid/B759BDE0E43DFB7F80256F43007634DC.

Kermani F. (2004), 'France Fights for its Pharma Future', *Inpharm*, 20 May at: http://www.inpharm.com/External/InpH/1,,1-3-0-0-inp_intelligence_art-0-196232,00.html.

Loriol, M. (2002), 'Quand l'observance religieuse influe sur l'observance médicale', 9 March at: http://www.moniteurpharmacies.com.

OECD (2003), 'OECD Health Data 2003 Show Health Expenditures at an All-time High', Organization for Economic Co-operation and Development at: http://www.oecd.org.

Maillard, C. (2003), 'Les Français et leurs médicaments' at: http://www.33doc.pro.com

Pharmaceutiques (2002), 'Les enjeux de la santé', 22 March at:. http://.pharmaceutiques.com

Part 3
Building for Success

Part 3 considers compliance from the start in the design, formulation and branding of health technology interventions (medicines), clinical trials, use of all possible resources including medical science liaison staff in the clinic and the use of technology to aid compliance with global examples, in particular from Japan and the United States.

CHAPTER 6

Building in Compliance from the Start

Janice MacLennan

As a pharmaceutical marketing consultant, a large part of the work that I am involved in concerns the formulation of strategy for the commercialization of new medicines. A key part of the strategy formulation is finding the best fit between the companies' asset and what the customer 'really' wants and/or needs. In the marketing world this is referred to as the 'brand positioning' or the 'brand concept'. Brands like Apple® and Harley Davidson® continue to maintain a very strong bond with their customers – this being because they clearly stand for something that unites people behind them.

'Best-practice' argues that the strategy formulation process should start prior to product decision with the intention of having an agreed strategy at the point of the go/no-go decision. This allows the company to shape the development programme so that it supports the brand strategy.

All too often, the brand strategy is developed with the physician as the primary target. Although this is appropriate when we are thinking of initiating the prescription, in my view, when it comes to driving compliance, the patient's attachment to the brand is of equal, if not more importance.

In this chapter, I explore the idea that a strong brand has the potential to drive patient adherence and, in so doing, influence patient compliance. First, I briefly discuss the difference between compliance and adherence. I then go on to review the extent to which the industry is succeeding with patient compliance with the intention of highlighting the issue. I then consider why this issue might exist. At this point I switch to my proposed solution: building a strong brand and shifting the focus to gaining patients' adherence and loyalty, rather than focusing on compliance.

COMPLIANCE VERSUS ADHERENCE

Compliance involves an involuntary act of submission to authority, whereas adherence refers to a voluntary act of subscribing to a point of view. The difference is not just semantic. The pharmaceutical industry needs to work both directly and indirectly (through the physician and others) to influence the patient into becoming and remaining committed to good self-care.

How big is the problem of poor patient compliance?

Given its size and importance, relatively little research has been conducted to quantify the scale of the poor compliance problem. However, the studies that have been done suggest that the extent of compliance varies widely and is highly drug- and patient-specific. It has been estimated that:

- in the United States, approximately one-third of patients take all of their medicine, one-third take 'some' and one-third take none at all (Hayes, 1989)
- approximately 125 000 people in the United States die annually due to non-compliance (Smith, 1989)
- over 50 per cent of prescriptions are taken incorrectly (NCIPE, n.d.)
- 10 per cent of all hospital admissions are due to patients taking their drugs incorrectly (Schering Report IX, 1987; Oregon Department of Human Resources, 1981).

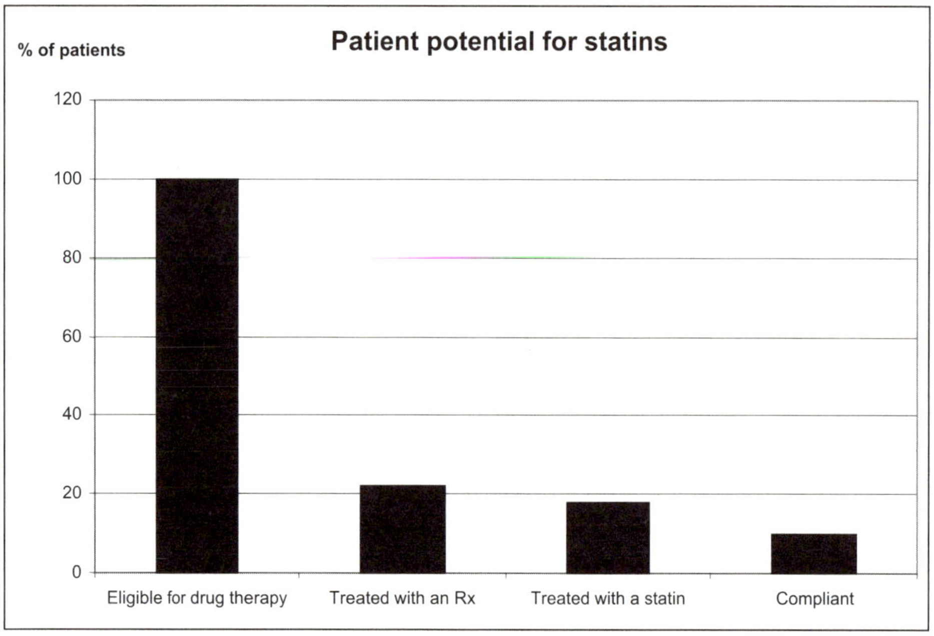

Note: Rx = prescription medicine.

Figure 6.1 The revenue potential associated with driving improvements in compliance

Patient non-compliance represents significant lost revenue to the pharmaceutical industry. According to Datamonitor (2003), patient non-compliance costs the pharmaceutical industry in excess of US$30 billion per year, patients suffer in terms of loss of quality of life, while the national health services also incur costs due to the consequences of patient non-compliance such as increased cardiovascular disease, and so forth.

Consider statins as an example (Roner, 2003). If you start with 100 per cent of the patient population who might be available and suitable for this drug therapy across multiple countries, on average only 22 per cent of those eligible patients get a prescription in the first place – and only 18 per cent of those are in fact on statins. But, more worryingly, only 10 per cent of patients are actually compliant. (Just one in three patients persists with statins after a year, and only one in eight after five years.) This means that, with statins alone, there is a 90 per cent gap for the industry to target (see Figure 6.1). And this is for a therapeutic area where the clinical benefits are already evident after just two years' therapy.

Such a significant lost opportunity should be seriously and continuously considered in all aspects of the business from research and development to commercialization and beyond.

Why do we see such low levels of compliance?

Several studies have looked at the factors leading to poor compliance and many of them relate to either poor, or even lack of, communication between the primary care physician and patient. Most patients feel unable to voice all their concerns to their doctor. One of the most common unvoiced concerns is fear and worry about the side-effects and/or safety of medication. These concerns have been elevated by the amount of press coverage surrounding drug withdrawals such as Vioxx. Other factors that have been shown to have an impact on compliance include:

- the nature of the treatment
- the characteristics of the patient, and
- the type of illness.

Although each of these factors is important in its own right, the nature of the treatment and the behaviour of the doctor are the most relevant when it comes to building a strong brand and gaining the patient's adherence and loyalty to this brand.

Let us begin with the nature of the treatment. Three factors determine the extent to which the nature of the treatment affects compliance. These are:

1. the patient's understanding of, and conviction as to, the potential benefit of the treatment
2. the complexity of the treatment regimen, and
3. any adverse effects associated with the regimen.

Typically the complexity of the regimen concerns both the frequency of administration and the number of drugs and/or formulations prescribed. The extent to which adverse reactions influence the patient's adherence to therapy tends to be related to the potential benefit (as perceived by the patient) of successfully completing the course of medication.

How does the behaviour of the doctor influence adherence? Interestingly, doctors and patients look at compliance through different lenses. While doctors value compliance and take it to be a necessary factor in treatment, patients value convenience, money, cultural beliefs, habits and image – any number of factors that may take precedence over the proposed treatment plan. A healthy dialogue on the benefit of treatment with the physician is a key component in driving adherence. The expectation that the patient will 'surrender' to the medical model is a central problem and is the reason why a compliance mindset generally doesn't work.

An International Osteoporosis Foundation survey conducted by IPSOS Health among 500 post-menopausal patients over 60 years in age and 500 doctors in France, Germany, Italy, Spain and the UK from January to April 2005, reveals that 34 per cent of those women interviewed either were not fully aware of the benefits of the medication or wrongly thought that there were no benefits at all (IOF, 2005). This suggests poor physician–patient dialogue.

HOW AND WHERE DOES THE STRENGTH OF THE BRAND IMPACT ON COMPLIANCE?

In the first instance, we need to agree what a brand is. A brand is not the physical object; it is what is sitting in the customer's head. Similarly, branding is not what happens on the page, but what goes on in the customer's head.

The 'brand concept' is the set of associations that a company would like people to hold about the brand so as to differentiate it from other marketplace offerings. In other words, it refers to the specific positioning of the brand in a competitive marketplace. The brand concept is derived from an analysis of the marketplace, competitors, the company's strengths, the product's differential advantages, target-market customers' needs or desired benefits and so on.

Strong brands tend to generate more customer loyalty. When I use the word 'customer', I am referring to the healthcare provider and the patient. I exclude the payer in this instance, because I think that it is unreasonable to expect a payer to be 'loyal' towards any one brand.

Brand loyalty is the extent to which the customer remains faithful to the brand over time. Strong commitment to a pharmaceutical brand is revealed by several behaviours. I am highlighting the behaviours which are relevant when talking about compliance - namely:

1. the physician taking the time to convince the patient of the benefit of treatment and, in so doing, counsel the patient on the importance of compliance;
2. the patient's continuing willingness to take the brand as prescribed in order to achieve the desired outcome;

3. the patient and/or the physician resisting substitution of the brand for a competitor's product;
4. trust in the brand – the patient and/or physician continuing to support the brand even during a brand crisis, public relations (PR) disaster or other brand mishap.

The importance of brand loyalty is highlighted by the discovery that the cost of gaining new customers is five times the cost of retaining existing ones. In the transparent markets of today, loyalty is not blind. It must be earned and continue to be earned. This is where branding (that is, the activities used to build the associations which establish that emotional attachment to the brand) has such a key role to play.

The current focus of the branding effort and possible future changes

Despite the often obvious value of a brand, there remain signs that the brand-building process is started, all too often, too late and emphasizes brand identity at the expense of other branding initiatives.

Today – cosmetic branding?

My experience with new product launches suggests that in many companies there is a disconnect between their product development process and the realities of the marketplace.

It is interesting to note that where there is evidence of investing in a pre-launch initiative to build the brand, it is happening two to three years before launch and is typically executed through branding guidelines. The branding guidelines focus on brand identity. The result? Every aspect of the brand's physical identity is regulated. Adherence to the guidelines is compulsory.

Conspicuous by their absence are any of the other dimensions that go into building a strong brand, and specifically nothing about the importance of the patient's emotional attachment to the brand and how this is intended to drive better compliance.

To too many people, the visual brand identity is the embodiment of the whole brand. Whilst the brand's identity encourages recognition and recall, it does not, in itself, communicate what the brand stands for and therefore has little impact on compliance.

Tomorrow – strategic branding?

The brand's role in the realm of pharmaceutical marketing has to change dramatically. Developing a brand involves devising and implementing a way by which to deliver a benefit to its customers. The brand concept will direct the development of the product, and services will be designed to support this benefit.

The new and strategic role of branding will remould the concept of branding. Brand-building will involve creating a system that, on the one hand, makes promises and arouses anticipations and, on the other hand, delivers and realizes the promises that it makes. In this way, it will forge that important emotional attachment.

Loyalty takes time. It requires cumulative positive experiences for people to identify with, or even bond with, a brand. Twenty-first century branding will require that the industry attends to the total brand experience, one that encompasses all messages, all channels, all touch points, with the customer as the guiding principle.

A large part of the brand-building experience when striving for loyalty is the patient experience. The challenge facing the pharmaceutical industry is to create a relationship between the patient and the brand by offering a customer-centric brand experience and then delivering this great brand experience time after time, from start to end.

One of the most critical steps: finding out why people do what they do

Strong brands understand customers in general and their orientation to the brand in particular. This means that, in order to 'build in compliance from the start', insight is needed. Insight is at the heart of brand development and life-cycle management.

Knowing what a valuable insight looks like and understanding how to leverage it is not easy, which is why it has the potential to create so much additional value. Over the years we have learnt that ideas are only as good as the insight they are founded on. Having lots of ideas is great, but unless they resonate with the customer, and are aligned to the brand concept they are unlikely to add much value.

A great example of a brand revitalized on the basis of insight is that of Cipramil®. The Lundbeck team used market research not as the basis for decision-making but as a starting point to develop customer insight.

They obtained the following insight: anti-depressants are perceived as '*effective but not tolerated*' and communicating an anti-depressant as 'clean' means '*not effective*' This helped them decide that the Cipramil brand needed to stand for anti-depression, not anti-patient, and to build the brand concept around 'uncomplicated efficacy'.

'Uncomplicated' is a great brand value because it has meaning to both the physician and the patient and it has real potential to drive patient compliance. Here is how:

- 'Uncomplicated', reinforced through product attributes such as dosing frequency and good toleration, will lead to better compliance.
- The ease of accessibility to the information associated with Cipramil further reinforces the concept of 'uncomplicated'.

If my theory is correct, consistently delivering against its brand promise – 'uncomplicated efficacy' – should lead to better patient compliance with this anti-depressant when compared with its competitive set.

BRANDING STRATEGIES WITH THE POTENTIAL TO DRIVE SUPPORT ADHERENCE AND THEREBY IMPROVE PATIENT COMPLIANCE

As we have discussed, the emotional attachment of patients to the brand is critical. To get this attachment we have to earn their trust. This has two broad strategic implications:

1. getting the brand concept right – that is, promising something that is relevant, distinctive and that we are able to deliver;
2. being guided by our brand concept when choosing the branding strategies.

The implementation of branding strategies affects the patient's brand perceptions, defined as the set of salient associations linked to the brand name in the customer's mind. If a company has been successful in its branding tactics via integrated medical–marketing communications, the perceptions that consumers hold of the brand will be the same as the brand concept. The following perceptions are the most important:

- *Brand image clarity.* The physician needs to be able to articulate clearly and concisely what prescribing the pharmaceutical brand is going to do for the patient and how it is different from other brands in the category. This will facilitate the physician–patient dialogue.
- *Belief in the brand.* At the same time, when the patients believe what the brand stands for, when they believe that it is responsive to their core need, and when they trust it, they will be far more likely to take it as prescribed.
- *Brand responsiveness.* This is the extent to which the brand is perceived to satisfy customers' important needs, particularly in relation to other brands in the category.
- *Brand trust.* This is the extent to which the brand is perceived as following through on promised claims and working in a way that is in the best interests of its customers.

Driving adherence

Patient empowerment programmes

The move away from the 'blanket' educational approach to more personalized patient communications is proving to be a most effective approach to strengthening the bond with the patient and thereby boosting patient adherence, but the cost of such a strategy is often seen as prohibitive.

Empowerment programmes designed to help the patient become an informed decision-maker and to shift the responsibility for managing the disease from the physician to the patient are proving to be successful. In a controlled trial in patients with diabetes, the empowerment programme was found to result in significant improvements in patients' perceptions of their ability to provide effective self-care, their attitudes towards living with diabetes and their metabolic control (Anderson *et al.*, 1995).

A great example of an empowerment programme that helps patients take responsibility

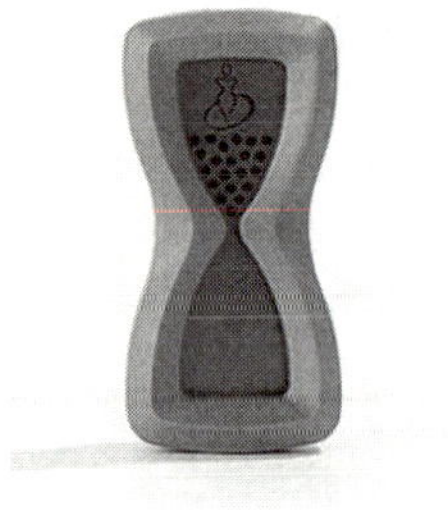

The NuvaTime reminder

The NuvaRing product website offers medication reminders for patients transitioning from once-daily to once-monthly therapy.

Figure 6.2 The NuvaTime reminder

for their treatment and, in so doing, impacts on patient compliance is that implemented by Nuvaring® (see Figure 6.2).

Other examples of successful patient empowerment programmes which drive adherence to therapy include those provided by:

- Betaseron® – a drug treatment for multiple sclerosis. MSPathways.com provides access to extensive support services for patients undergoing treatment with Betaseron.
- Levitra® – a drug treatment for erectile dysfunction. Levitra's product website offers patients the option of filling prescriptions online, overcoming the 'embarrassment factor' that may prevent some patients from filling their prescriptions.

Improving sales force effectiveness

According to InPharm, although the top 40 pharmaceutical companies have doubled the size of their sales forces in the past five years, prescribing has increased by only 15 per cent. The discrepancy between growth in sales force size and growth in prescribing is making sales force effectiveness the top challenge among pharmaceutical sales managers. The winners will be those that succeed in using the sales force to help create the strong brand. The sales force therefore need to understand how and where they can contribute to developing a strong bond between the brand(s) that they are selling and their different customers.

Most physicians live in fear of salespeople with PowerPoint presentations – salespeople who spend their time explaining why their products are so great and why their company is wonderful, and almost no time listening and learning what physicians, as customers, need and want. The key is to listen, understand and respond. There is a need for an ongoing exchange in which the industry listens carefully to its customers, understands what they are saying and responds appropriately to fulfil their desires.

Remember, where physicians are convinced of the benefits of a brand and believe that the company is doing what it can to facilitate compliance, they will take the time to discuss the benefit of the therapy (and therefore the importance of adherence) with their patients.

The final ingredient that binds a customer to the brand in a lasting relationship is dialogue. An ongoing dialogue needs to exist between the company, physician and patient, and the industry needs to take the lead in making this happen. The following suggestions, based on the most recent findings of the communications research that I have been involved in, offer some ways in which the industry can take this lead:

- Understand the patient's language – and use it. Introduce this language to the physician with a view to helping them strengthen the physician–patient dialogue and establish a rapport.
- Shift from scientific language to the language of feelings: show the patients that we care by expressing feelings about progress, problems and so on.
- Base treatment goals on an insight into both the physicians' and patients' goals.
- Support patient learning: provide the patient with, or direct them to, the information that they are seeking

Supporting adherence

The value of drug delivery systems

Drug delivery is focusing on developing more 'user-friendly' dosage forms of medicines with the ultimate aim of increasing dosing convenience for the patient. This may involve reducing dosage frequency or developing an oral formulation of a drug that is traditionally given by injection or creating an oral formulation that is easier to take (for example, 'fast-melt' tablets that dissolve in the mouth or effervescent sachets that produce pleasant-tasting medicines).

From the physician's perspective, providing medicine in a more acceptable format is desirable in terms of improving patient compliance. From the patient's perspective, convenience helps adherence to the treatment programme.

Nowhere have the benefits of this type of branding strategy been more evident than in asthma with the introduction of the Advair® / Seretide® brand. At the core of the brand concept is the idea of 'freeing' the patients from their asthma. The Advair/Seretide brand does this in a number of ways, as illustrated in Figure 6.3.

Combining oral medications is generally thought to be a solution to patient non-compliance. The major drug companies such as Pfizer, Merck and Schering-Plough have begun to market combination drugs that treat different facets of a single condition. Prime examples include Merck's Vytorin®, a cholesterol-lowering drug, and Pfizer's Caduet®, a combination of a calcium channel blocker and a lipid-lowering agent.

The great thing about drug delivery is that the benefits have meaning to both the

1. The inhaler contains two products in one inhaler, ensuring that the patient gets both the inhaled corticosteroid and the long-acting bronchodilator every time they take their medication, leading to better patient outcomes

2. The 'anti-inflammatory' agent is delivered through the inhaled route, thus overcoming some of the concerns with the side-effect/safety issues associated with oral corticosteroids.

3. It has a fixed dosing schedule (one or two puffs twice daily), which helps the patient remember to take their medication.

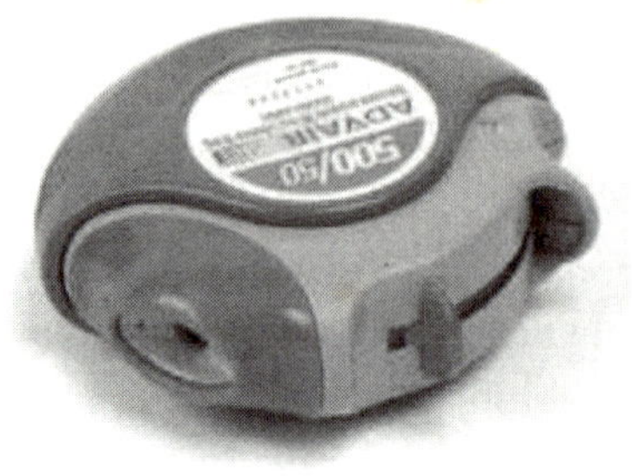

Image reproduced by kind permission of GlaxoSmithKline.

Figure 6.3 The Advair/Seratide branding strategy

physician and the patient and so can be used to establish the desired emotional attachment with both parties.

DRUG SAFETY PROGRAMMES

In the light of recent high-profile drug withdrawals, most companies today will be proactively developing strategies to manage risk and enhance patient safety. These should not be considered separately but integrated into the overall branding strategy to ensure that it is aligned to the brand concept.

The biggest barrier? Gaining the patient's trust

Although we can easily recognize the importance of trust, the bad press that the pharmaceutical industry attracts makes it increasingly difficult to build this bond. Below are some tips that may help you.

- *Demonstrate commitment.* When customers know that you are committed to them, they will begin to trust you. Ideally, you want to demonstrate your commitment by listening and responding to what your customers are saying.
- *Be consistent.* If your brand is trying to say that you do something, do it and do it well. Repeat this process over and over.
- *Honesty is the best policy.* You cannot deceive your customers and expect to be successful in the long term. How your company responds to legitimate customer concerns can make or break you.

Tylenol® is universally applauded for the way in which it handled the tampering scare of the 1980s. The company responded quickly and appropriately to the crisis by publicly addressing the problem, pulling 264 000 bottles off of store shelves, and later reintroducing a safer, more tamperproof package for their product. The Tylenol brand is stronger today because of the way in which this crisis was handled.

THE BOTTOM LINE

There is no escaping the role of the *brand* in the drive to get patients to, and support patients with, adherence to their medication and thereby improving compliance. Developing the brand–customer relationship is so important – either you make the customer experience or it gets made without you.

To create a successful brand-customer relationship you must develop a compelling value proposition and brand identity, as well as having the ability to listen and respond appropriately to evolve your product's offering to meet customers' needs and desires from the earliest opportunity.

Good branding, then, means doing a lot of things right: identifying a good brand concept at the outset; formulating a good development and life-cycle management plan; and designing a good marketing mix that creates a strong and clear brand image, creates trust and makes the different customers feel that the brand is responsive to their different needs. It means thinking strategically – using good sense about your brand's core meaning and thinking about how to forge that emotional bond with a view to building in 'adherence' from the start.

The following facts are worth considering:

- When it comes to compliance it is recognized that everyone benefits from better patient compliance because better compliance equals better efficacy which, in turn, means better patient outcomes. But, compliance is the wrong mindset – adherence is better.
- We are loyal to certain brands for the same reason that we are loyal to our friends, because we like them (easy to take), they do not let us down (safety and efficacy), and we share the same outlook (the desire for a positive outcome).
- Each and every product-related decision that is taken during the product's life cycle has the potential to contribute to, or undermine, the strength of the brand.

- Deriving customer insight is a capability. Knowing what a valuable insight looks like and understanding how to leverage it is not easy. The industry lacks this capability. Be prepared to work with people outside the industry to develop this capability.
- Building 'adherence' thinking into product development programmes requires attention to medication satisfaction, patient preferences and clinical and economic outcomes, as well as quality of life and health status considerations.

REFERENCES

Anderson, R.M., Funnell, M.M., Butler, P.M., Arnold, M.S., Fitzgerald, J.T. and Feste, C.C. (1995), 'Patient Empowerment: Results of a Randomized Controlled Trial', *Diabetes Care*, **18**(7), pp. 943–49.

Datamonitor (2003), 'Improving Patient Compliance: Utilizing Online and Mobile Compliance Tools', 16 July 2003.

Hayes, R.B. (1989), *NCPIE Prescription Month*, October 1989, p. 7.

IOF (2005), 'The Adherence Gap: Why Osteoporosis Patients Don't Continue With Treatment: A European Report Highlighting the Gap between the Beliefs of People with Osteoporosis and the Perceptions of their Physicians, International Osteoporosis Foundation, available at: http://www.osteofound.org/publications/adherence_gap_report.html

NCPIE National Council for Patient Information and Education (n.d.) at: http://www.talkaboutrx.org/med (downloaded 2005).

Oregon Department of Human Resources (1981), *A Study of Long-Term Care in Oregon with Emphasis on the Elderly*, March, Oregon: Oregon Department of Human Resources.

Rona, L. (2005), 'Making Patient Compliance Part of the SFE Mix', Eyeforpharma, 14 April at: http://www.eyeforpharma.com/search.asp?news=45650.

Schering Report IX (1987), *The Forgetful Patient: The High Cost of Improper Patient Compliance*, Falls Church, VA: Healthcare Compliance Packaging Council.

Smith, D. (1989), 'Compliance Packaging: A Patient Education Tool', *American Pharmacy*, **NS29**(2), February , pp. 49–53.

CHAPTER 7

Formulating for Compliance Success

Dr Akira Kusai, PhD

The rapid development and provision of the right products to medical institutions and patients is a key role of the pharmaceutical industry. The 'right product' will depend on a number of circumstances which will affect how appropriate a product is to a particular patient. This includes satisfying an unmet medical need amongst patients, providing patients with prompt relief from a condition in a manner which results in fewer side-effects than their currently available treatment, improving their quality of life, providing a more patient-friendly product or developing a novel concept to treat the patients' condition. Furthermore, the company may benefit if its product opens up a new market.

It is within this context that more attention has been paid to 'compliance'. Compliance has become a key factor during product development and during launch as it relates to a product being perceived as 'right' by patients.

Japan is the third major regional pharmaceutical market in the world and, given its importance, in this chapter I would like to discuss some of the compliance issues relevant to the market from the perspective of the pharmaceutical industry. The chapter will discuss a variety of dosage forms such as solids, parenterals and non-invasive forms for the systemic treatment of disease, as well as related technologies, and link these to patient compliance. Several issues concerning packaging will also be mentioned. The field of compliance is complex and, in order to retain focus on the above points, I will not cover areas such as the verification of patient prescriptions and educating patients on how to use their medicines.

No doubt many of the points will appear familiar to those with experience in the USA and Europe, but some are considered specific to Japan and it is these points that I hope to also bring to the attention of readers. The reasons for these country-specific factors partly result from traditional Japanese pharmaceutical habits, whilst others relate to specific dispensing skills in this country.

CHOICE OF DOSAGE FORM

Solid dose forms

Oral dosage forms are quite common because they are easy to handle, manufacture, dispense and administer. Figure 7.1 shows the constitution of oral dosage forms in Japan, the USA and Germany. Tablets are more common than capsules. However, granules and powders (including fine granules) are a noticeably characteristic feature of the Japanese market and these will be discussed in greater detail later.

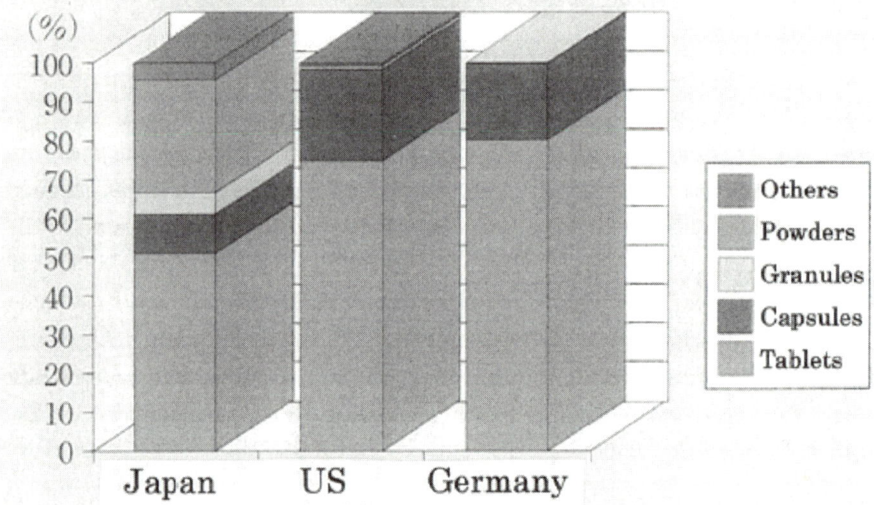

Source: Nagata (2004).

Figure 7.1 Types of oral dosage forms: comparison between Japan, the USA and Germany

In this section, a comparison is made between the market for tablets and capsules, and there will be a discussion of issues relating to dosage form design. This includes areas such as controlled release, oral dissolving tablets, granules and fine granules, and activities carried out at dispensing counters such as the grinding of tablets, splitting tablets into half, and single-dose packaging.

Tablets or capsules

Tablets and capsules are representative examples of solid drug forms. As Figure 7.1 shows, in Japan, sales of tablets outstrip sales of capsules by a ratio of five to one – a greater ratio than in the USA and Germany (Nagata, 2004). The preference of patients for tablets which they consider easy to swallow partly explains this observation. However, the trend towards tablets can also be explained by the physical properties of typical new drug candidates and the willingness of Japanese pharmaceutical scientists to explore this formulation strategy. New drug candidates tend to have low solubility, so in order to improve their dissolution properties, as well as their manufacturing potential, granules tend to be prepared with excipients using wet granulation methods (Yakahashi *et al.*, 1998). Fluidized bed granulators and high-shear mixers are commonly found in Japanese industrial plants. Once the granules have been prepared, tablets are manufactured through a compression process whereas capsules are filled with granules. In general the compression rate for tablets is much faster than filling capsules. In addition, capsules are rather more expensive than other common excipients that are used for solid dosage forms.

It is unclear as yet what the future trends will be regarding the ratio of tablets to capsules over the next decade in Japan. One issue that will have an impact is the concern over bovine spongiform encephalopathy (BSE). Capsule manufactures are struggling to find an alternative supply for gelatine, rather than relying on the traditional bovine sources. This change is taking place even though several measures are in place to check bovine sources and processes are being developed to completely deactivate prions (Otsuka, 2001; Okada, 1999). Pork-derived and fish-derived gelatine are being explored and use is being made of polymers such as hydroxypropylmethylcellulose (HPMC) (Ogura *et al.*, 1999) and pullulan (Onuki, 2004). The use of polyvinyl acetate (PVA) for capsule shells is also now under development (Hoshi *et al.*, 2003). However, these tend to be even more charged materials than bovine gelatine capsules. The cost implications for alternative sources also need to be explored and their supply needs to be guaranteed.

It is possible that capsules will increase their market share as pharmaceutical companies try to develop their products as rapidly as possible. To do so, the drug candidates are simply dissolved or suspended in an oily base and filled into capsules in order to conduct Phase I and IIa human clinical studies (Hoshi *et al.*, 2003).

Identification: colour and shape of dosage forms

Pharmaceutical products should be easily identified and differentiated from other products. In the case of tablets, this is conducted through their shape, size and colour, marking by engraving and printing, and packaging. In the US market, tablets with a combination of unique shape and colour are on the market, and this not only helps to promote them, but also distinguishes them from competitors' products. In Japan, products tend to be identified primarily through colour and markings, although this may change in the future.

In Japan there is a belief that the optimal size for a tablet is between 7 and 8 mm in diameter (Sugihara, 1994) since it is thought that this size makes the tablet easy for the patient to hold and swallow. Japanese patients favour light colours, particularly white as it conveys the image of purity – that is, a product free from contaminants. However, many dispensing chemists actually prefer a darker colour because it increases the identification potential.

With respect to the marking on tablets, engraving is more common than printing. The former is often conducted at the time of compressing. Printing is considered to make it easier for a patient to differentiate products from those of competitors.

In the case of capsules, colour again plays a major role in identification, although printing and packaging are used to enhance the product features. Once again, Japanese patients favour lighter colour capsules to those with darker colours.

Drug combinations

Drug combinations – or 'drug combos' – can serve as a useful means to increase patient compliance. There are a number of famous historical examples of this approach such as levodopa/carbidopa for Parkinson's disease, sulfa/trimethoprim for human immunodeficiency virus (HIV) infection and oestrogen/progesterone as oral contraceptives. The current trend in combination drugs is related to lifestyle diseases and areas such as hypertension, hyperlipidaemia and diabetes. Examples launched or under clinical development in the USA and Europe include ARB (angiotensin II antagonist)/diuretics,[1] statin/cholesterol absorption inhibitors,[2] statin/ARB[3] and insulin sensitizer/liver gluconeogenesis inhibitors.[4]

A drug combo contains several active pharmaceutical ingredients (APIs) with the same or different pharmacological effects. There is an expectation in Japan that drug combos will enhance efficacy and have better adverse event profiles than the dosage forms containing only one API. An additional advantage is that drug combos effectively help patients to remember to take their medicines (when compared to them taking several kinds of monotherapy drugs at the same time) and avoids the risk of taking different medicines in the wrong amounts. The cheaper price for a drug combo (compared with buying two or more APIs separately) is also an attractive feature for patients.

For innovative pharmaceutical companies, there is less risk in developing a drug combo, because the side-effects of each API are well known. Furthermore, this has benefits in terms of life-cycle management (Ansell, 2005). Even if the patent for monotherapy has expired, the drug combo allows a company to gain further commercial advantage through a new product patent. This acts as a useful defence against generic manufacturers, whilst serving as an important improvement in the area of patient compliance.

Previously in Japan, there was a requirement that the manufacturer must show that a drug combo results in synergistic effects of its constituent products, rather than an additive effect. However, since Notification No. 03300001 was issued in March 2005,[5] the benefits of a drug combo in terms of improving patient compliance have been recognized.

1. Losartan/HCTZ (Merck & Co. Inc.), Olmesartan/HCTZ (Sankyo Pharma Inc.), Candesartan/HCTZ (Takeda Pharmaceuticals North America, Inc.) and so on.
2. Ezetimibe/Simvastatin (Schering–Plough Corporation/Merck & Co. Inc.).
3. Amlogipine besylate/Atorvastatin calcium (Pfizer Inc.).
4. Pioglitazon/Metformin (Takeda Pharmaceuticals North America, Inc.).
5. Notification No. 03300001 of ELD, PFBS, MHLW dated 30 March 2005.

Modified release

To maximize pharmacological activity and safety, dosage forms are developed by taking the disease characteristics, the patient's condition and the biopharmaceutical characteristics of candidates into consideration. For oral dosage forms, companies wish to deliver an appropriate amount of drug to the required site at the desired time. Thus, modified release techniques are considered to be a very important part of the development strategy for a product. Here three types of controlled drug delivery systems will be discussed – that is, rate-controlled release, time-controlled release and site-specific controlled release.

During the screening stage of new drug candidates, the absorption, distribution, metabolism and excretion (ADME) profile is one of the factors to be considered, as well as safety and pharmacological profiles. The estimation of half-life after administration to humans is crucial, as it directly affects how often the product will need to be administered each day. For oral candidates, once-daily dosing is considered ideal, although twice-daily dosing is also considered to be acceptable. When appropriate candidates are selected, formulations for the conventional solid dosage forms take preference. However, if dosing more than three times daily is estimated to be required, then great efforts are made to determine whether a once-daily or twice-daily dosage form can be developed through other means. Controlled release forms are prepared, such as matrix tablets, multi-pills, capsules, tablets coated with special microporous films and gel-forming tablets. Oily semi-solid matrix (capsules) (Seta *et al.*, 1988) and oral controlled absorption systems consisting of polyethylene oxide and polyethylene glycols as basic components (tablets) (Sako *et al.*, 1996; Sako, 1998) are examples of approaches invented in Japan.

Time-controlled release dosage forms behave as if they carry a timer function with them – after a predetermined interval post-administration, the dosage form promptly releases the APIs. This concept is often applied to pharmaceutical products that patients are expected to use during the night or during the early morning. In Japan this concept is considered suitable for pharmaceuticals used for treating diseases such as asthma, hypertension, rheumatism, and orthostatic hypotension. Techniques used to achieve this effect include membrane disruption, membrane dissolution, membrane peeling and the time-dependent change of membrane permeation. Some of the more innovative approaches invented in Japan include time-controlled explosion systems (Hata *et al.*, 1994), sigmoidal release systems (Narisawa *et al.*, 1994) and pulsatile tablets (Ishino *et al.*, 1992).

To target a product for release in the stomach, small intestine or large intestine requires site-specific control. Coating the core tablets with polymer films dissolved at gastric pH or enteric pH is the well-established procedure. In contrast, utilizing polymers that adhere to the gastric mucus, and azopolymers which are fragmented and dissolved by micro-organisms in the large intestine represent alternative yet novel approaches. Polymers such as carbopol (Akiyama *et al.*, 1993; Akiyama, 2001), chitosan (Kawashima, 2004) and azo-containing polyurethanes (Nishioka *et al.*, 1997) have been investigated in Japan.

Oral dissolving tablets

Oral dosage forms such as tablets and capsules tend to be administered with water. However, they are often not appropriate for elderly patients and children, who have difficulty in swallowing in the required manner. Thus oral dissolving tablets are good way of dealing with this problem (Tsushima, 2004). They are also useful for situations when a patient may not have access to water yet wishes to take the medicine. Currently, the oral dissolving tablet approach is being explored in Japan in a number of areas for both prescription and over-the-counter (OTC) drugs, such as tranquillizers, anti-nausea agents, anti-ulcer agents, anti-hypertension agents, anti-Alzheimer agents, anti-diabetes agents, drugs for car sickness and antacids.

Three processes are generally used to manufacture oral dissolving tablets:

1. moulding the wet granules followed by drying
2. compression of the dried granules into tablets, followed by moistening with aqueous vapour or alcohol and drying, and
3. filling the solution or suspension into pockets followed by drying or lyophilization.

Several Japanese pharmaceutical companies have developed their own technologies in this area. Potentially, the market size is large and so there is a high level of competition between pharmaceutical companies to develop oral dissolving tablet formulations in addition to conventional tablet products.

In Japan, oral dissolving tablets are classified as tablets according to the general rules of preparation. When such tablets are developed as additional products, companies must prove that they are not absorbed through oral mucus membranes and that they are bioequivalent to the conventional tablets launched. As such, they must meet the following conditions:

1. The pharmacokinetics of oral dissolving tablets administered with water must be comparable with those obtained from reference tablets administered with water.
2. The pharmacokinetics of oral dissolving tablets administered without water must be comparable with those obtained from reference tablets administered with water.

The first point must be satisfied in all cases; if the second point is valid, a company may state in the package insert that the product can be taken without water.

Fine granules and granules

Granules are part of the manufacturing process of tablets or capsules in the USA and Europe. However, in Japan they often also represent the final dosage forms to a greater degree than in other countries. The tradition of Chinese herbal medicines, which are administered as powders, has heavily influenced the preference of the Japanese patient for powders and granules as a major pharmaceutical dosage form. To improve flow and dusting properties, products are formulated as granules and fine granules. They are manufactured mainly using a wet granulation method through a combination of a high-shear mixer and an extruder, or a fluid bed granulator. They are also prepared by a dry granulation method using a roll granulator or by slugging. According to *The Pharmacopoeia of Japan* (2001), the definitions are as follows:

> *Granules:* All the granules should pass through a No.10 (1700mm) sieve, with not more than 5% of total granules remaining on a No.12 (1400mm) sieve, and not more than 15% of total granules passing through a No. 42 (355mm) sieve.
> *Fine Granules:* All the powders should pass through a No.18 (850mm) sieve, with not more than 5% of total granules remaining on a No.30 (500mm) sieve. Powders with not more than 10% of total passing through a No.200 (75mm) sieve may be described as Fine Granules.

Patients – particularly those children and elderly patients who have difficulty swallowing tablets or capsules – and dispensing pharmacists generally welcome such improved physical properties for a product. Indeed, these dosage forms are suitable even for adults when a large powder mixture of higher strength, such as 2g, is required. To mask the bitter taste of granules or fine granules, film coatings are used and/or flavours added. In the USA and Europe, flavoured granules are prescribed as suspensions at dispensing counters. However in Japan, although granules are occasionally dispensed in this form, they are generally dispensed as unit-dose sachets. The patient adds water to create a suspension just before dosing, or the product is administered in the granular form itself, accompanied by water.

Oral gel products

Oral gel products, like those shown in Figure 7.2, may offer a useful alternative for patients who cannot easily swallow tablets, capsules and even granules (Tsushima, 2004). In extreme cases, some patients cannot even drink water, but may nevertheless still be

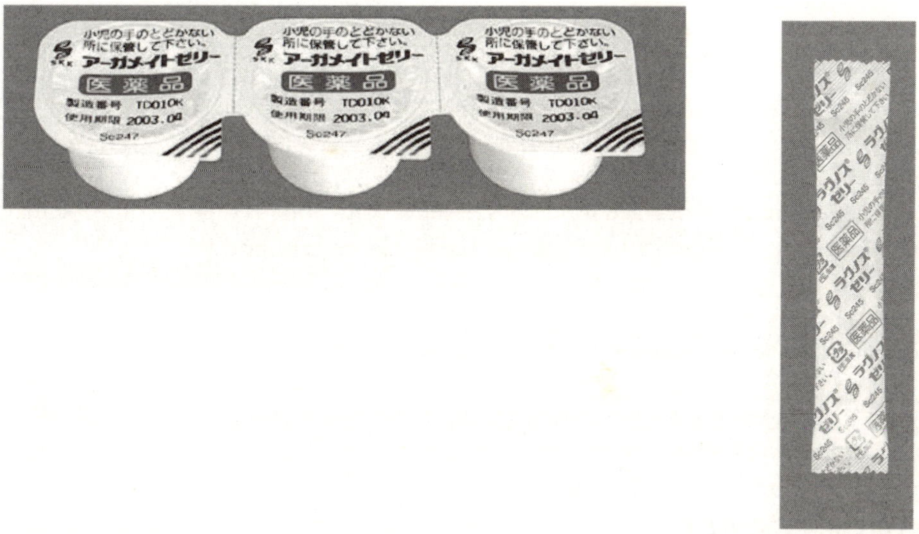

Reproduced by kind permission of Teikoku Medix Co. Ltd. and Sanwa Kagaku Kenktyysho Co., Ltd.

Figure 7.2 Oral gel products

able to drink or swallow viscous solutions. Agar powders at a concentration of around 1 per cent can play a role in enhancing the viscosity of aqueous solutions or suspensions.

Although it is not considered to be a pharmaceutical product in its own right, agar powder is often sold in Japan as a gelling agent and it is used to thicken foods for elderly bedridden patients at mealtimes or when drugs need to be administered with water.

Unit-dose packs of oral solution or suspension

Syrups are usually prescribed in Japan in multi-dose packages to cover several days of treatment. However, many patients have difficulties in using the dosing vessel correctly. Furthermore, this approach does leave open the possibility of contamination by micro-organisms. To circumvent these problems new unit-dose oral solutions or suspensions have been launched onto the market (Tsushima, 2004).

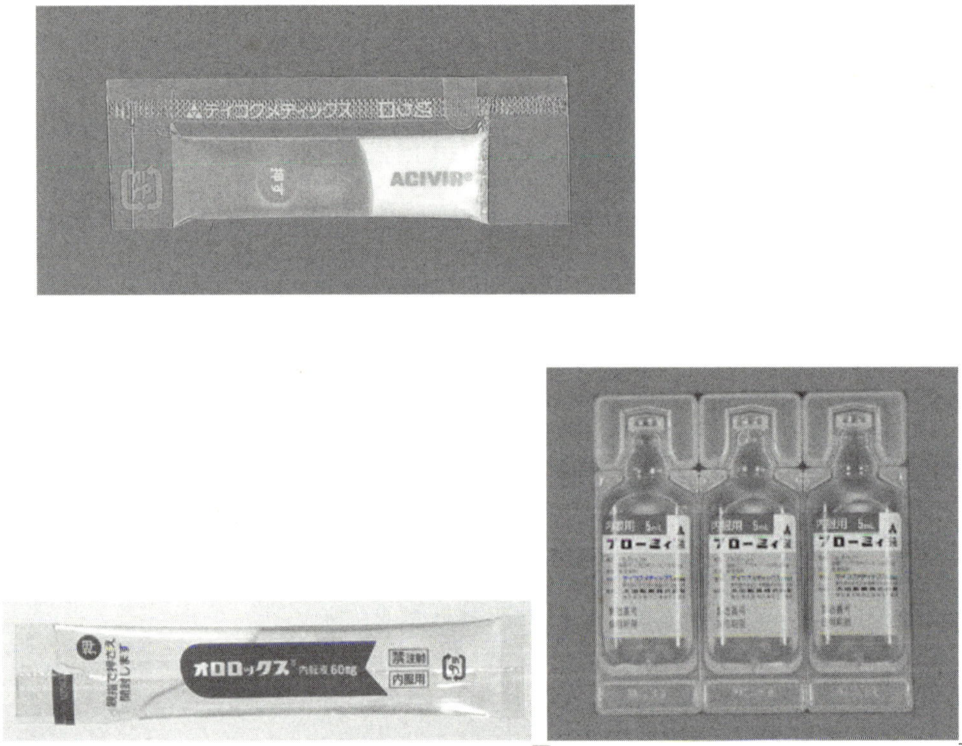

Reproduced by kind permission of Teikoku Medix Co. Ltd.

Figure 7.3 Unit-dose pack of oral solution and suspension

PARENTERALS

In this section, topics related to dosage form design, self-injection devices such as needle-less injection devices and painless needles, kit products and packaging materials are discussed in relation to patient compliance.

Controlled release

Even when administered by an experienced physician, most people dislike injections, and only when the condition is serious are patients willing to bear the pain of regular injections. Therefore, one way of improving patient compliance is to reduce the frequency of injection – for example, through the use of depot dosage forms. A common method is to use a biodegradable polymer, such as polylactic acid-polyglycolic acid copolymer (PLGA) to prepare microspheres containing active ingredients. Once injected intramuscularly, they degrade slowly to release the active ingredients. For example, microspheres containing luteinizing hormone-releasing hormone (LHRH) analogues as once a month dosage forms and once every three-month dosage forms were invented in Japan and are now marketed globally (Okada, 1997, 1998). Atelocollagen pellets of proteins for direct injection and implantation into muscle are at the preclinical and clinical stages of development (Sano *et al.*, 1998, 2003).

Incompatibility tests

Another way of improving compliance is to reduce the number of injections required. This can be achieved by administering several injections together by mixing before the injection procedure. When developing a new product for injection, such an approach can be tested in relation to other injectable products, including infusions. This information is included in the New Drug Application (NDA) submission and is provided to the medical doctors and pharmacists (Nagai, 1999).

Product kits and pre-filled syringes

Product kits are also a useful means of improving patient compliance. According to the Drug Approval and Licensing Procedures in Japan (1998, pp. 349–51), product kits are defined as products consisting of a drug and a medical device or two or more drugs for a single administration, which are intended to facilitate drug administration procedures and prevent contamination with bacteria or foreign matter when drugs are prepared for administration in hospitals. As illustrated in Figure 7.4, kits are classified into four types:

1. pre-filled syringe
2. two or more chamber type, which can be mixed or reconstituted just before administration (see Figure 7.5)
3. one chamber of already diluted or mixed drug
4. two drugs in separate containers, one of which is to be dissolved in the other at the time of use through a special connecting chamber.

Multichamber systems are manufactured with films consisting of two kinds of resins, one of which melts at a lower temperature than the other (Drug Approval and Licensing Procedures in Japan, 1998, pp. 349–51). When the chambers are constructed, the outside is heat-sealed at a high temperature sufficient to melt both resins, and the partition zones of each part are heat-sealed at the temperature in between. Thus when pressure is applied by hand, the weakest parts – that is, the partition parts – are detached, and the ingredients of each chamber can be mixed together, or reconstituted, ready for administration.

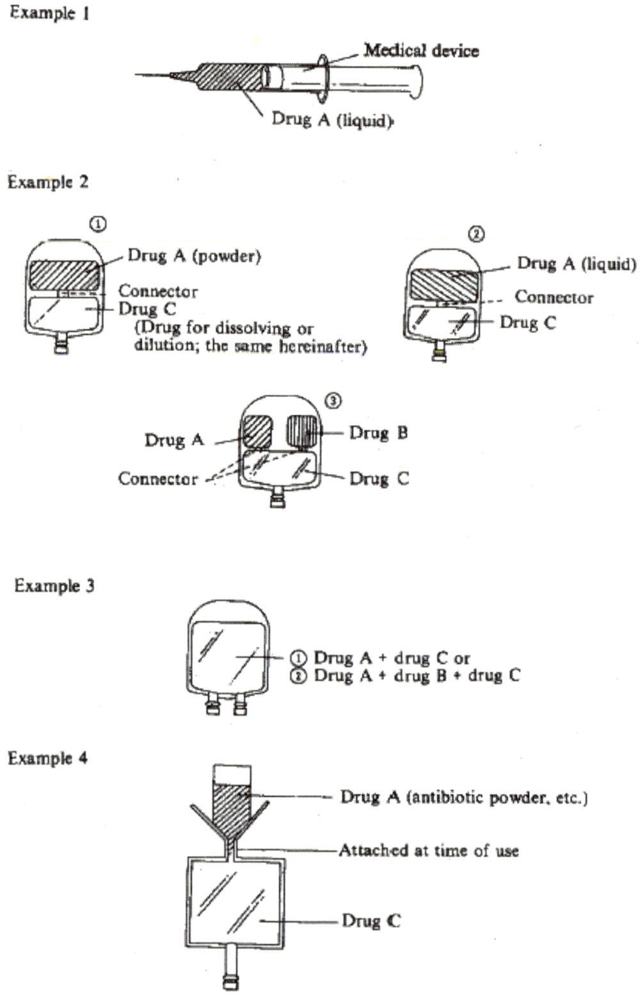

Figure 7.4 Four types of product kit

Product kits must be clearly labelled with the full name of the drugs, which should prevent medical administration errors at the time of dosing. The kits are useful in emergency situations as drugs may be readily administered without lengthy reconstitution or mixing. Contamination with bacteria and foreign matter such as glass fragments from ampoules and coatings from rubber stoppers is also prevented. Thus, all these facts in combination act to improve the scenario for patient compliance (Izumi, 1999; Kuroyama *et al.*, 1999a, 1999b; Hirayama *et al.*, 1999).

Self-injection devices, needle-less injection devices and painless needles

Self-injection devices

As mentioned above, people dislike injections given by doctors. Thus devices for self-injection are useful. Currently, insulin and growth hormone are examples of pharmaceuticals permitted for self-injection in Japan. They are administered subcutaneously. Identifiable ways of improving the patient compliance include measures to avoid the use of needles with the syringe or the development of painless needles.

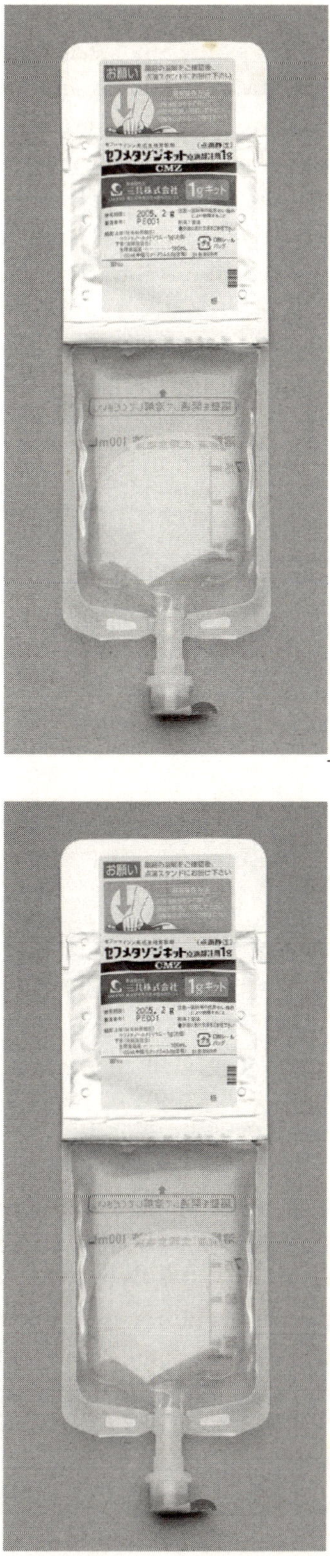

Reproduced by kind permission of Sankyo Co. Ltd.

Figure 7.5 Multichamber product kits

The first approach requires a 'needle-less' injection device. Shimaject^{TM}, illustrated in Figure 7.6 and invented and patented by the Shimadzu Corporation, a company with a well-established reputation for analytical equipment, and Twinjector II are examples of this approach that are available in Japan. Essentially, the high pressure stored in the device resulting from the spring is sufficient to inject the pharmaceutical subcutaneously. The tip size of the nozzle is 0.17mm, which is 0.08mm less than smallest needle available. When the injection is administered with this device, it causes less pain and less bleeding than conventional syringes employing needles. It is also worth noting the additional advantages of this approach. For example, the patient does not have to worry about accidentally leaving a broken needle at the injection site after the procedure and there is less chance of infection by micro-organisms. This device has been used in insulin self-injection kits in Japan since 2001.

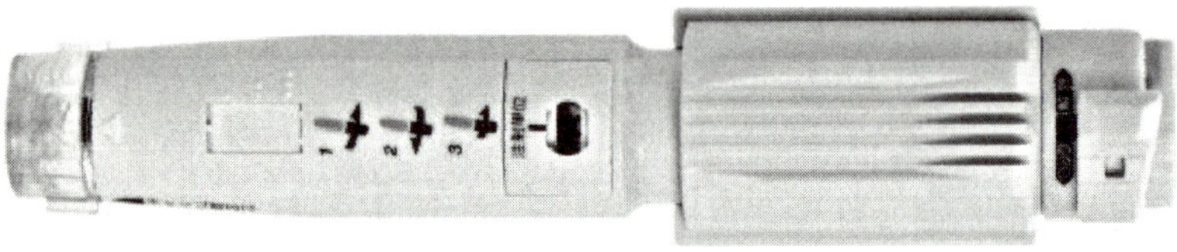

Reproduced by kind permission of Shimadzu Corporation

Figure 7.6 Shimaject^{TM}

Painless needles

Pen-type syringes are quite commonly used for self-injection worldwide. If they cause less pain, that can only be good news for patients for whom self-injection is unavoidable. Previously, advances in this area were slow, but it has recently been reported that the goal of developing painless needles is becoming more realistic (Asukura and Seino, 2004; *Asahi Shimbun*, 2005; *Nikkei Sangyo Shimbun*, 2005).

Interestingly, some of the approaches towards developing painless injection procedures have been based on examining the physiology of mosquitoes, as their presence is often not detected while they are obtaining blood from victims. As a result of this unusual approach, the needle diameter, from the bottom to the tip, has been gradually narrowed to a 33-gauge tip and a 28-gauge base. The outer diameter of the tip is 0.2mm and inner diameter is 0.1mm. These needles are not manufactured in the conventional manner, which involves the elongation of a stainless steel tube. Instead, a special technology used in metal sheet processing is now being applied. This provides the unique shape described above. Consequently, the inner needle surface is very smooth, which means that the injection solution can flow with less friction. It is reported that this needle will be launched in Japan within this year at an affordable price. Another benefit is that the manufacturing system is well suited to mass production. Such an approach is likely to find favour with patients.

TRANSMUCOUS DRUG DELIVERY OF SYSTEMIC TREATMENT

If the drugs that are parenterally administered for systemic treatment are delivered non-invasively, they can greatly improve patient compliance. In this section, dermal patches, inhalation approaches and nasal sprays are discussed.

Dermal patches

Plasters and cataplasms are often employed as dosage forms in Japan, especially to treat stiff shoulder, muscular aches and local inflammation. Traditionally, if people had such symptoms, they would collect medicinal herbs and rub them into the affected body parts. This historical approach has now been transformed into the modern plaster and cataplasm. Therefore, from a social perspective, Japanese patients are well accustomed to these dosage forms and are happy to use them.

Recently, dermal patches for systemic, rather than just local, treatment have been developed. Not only are they non-invasive and easily applied, but they also have the advantage that they avoid direct potential gastrointestinal damage and improve the compliance of elderly patients and children by controlling the blood concentration of the drug for several days – in other words, the continuous release of the desired systemic treatment can be attained (Onuki and Okabe, 2004). In addition, it is not only relatively straightforward for healthcare workers to determine whether or not the patches have been administered, but also to manage the patient, if adverse effects are observed, by simply removing the patch. At present, patches of nitroglycerin, estradiol, nicotine and scopolamine are available on the Japanese market.

Inhalations and nasal sprays

Due to the development of biotechnology, proteins can be prepared on a large scale and have thus become candidates to treat diseases. However their bioavailability makes them inappropriate for development as oral dosage forms, because of poor absorption through gastrointestinal membranes and poor gastrointestinal stability resulting from drastic pH changes and the presence of digestive enzymes. Thus injections are conventionally selected to solve these problems.

Recently, the lungs and nasal mucus membranes have been found to be suitable locations for the administration of systemic drugs, as they have better permeability profiles and possess fewer digestive enzymes (Morishita 2002; Todo *et al.*, 2002). Many Japanese pharmaceutical scientists have begun to focus on inhalation approaches and nasal sprays as alternative means of administering drugs. Several products are likely to appear on the Japanese market, but this will depend on how effectively pharmaceutical companies can collaborate with medical device manufacturers specializing in the delivery aspect of medicines.

NANOPARTICLES

When considering patient compliance, it is now impossible to neglect the field of nanoparticle technology. When nanoparticles of poorly soluble drugs are orally administered in submicron sizes, bioavailability is greatly improved, there tends to be less variability between patients and the ingestion of food generally has less effect on the treatment. Technologies used in this field include reducing particle size by means of a high-pressure homogenizer and crystallizing them from solvents (Liversidge, 2004; Rabinow, 2004).[6]

When the particles are reduced to submicron sizes, they can be injected intravenously in a suspended state with less surfactant and without any co-solvents. This inevitably enhances the chances of patient compliance.

The approach involving micelle-forming block polymers was invented in Japan (Kataoka, 2000). It consists of a hydrophilic polymer moiety (polyethyleneglycol) and a hydrophobic polymer moiety (poly-amino acid derivatives). Once dispersed in water, they spontaneously associate to form two-tier particles of 20 to 100nm, which consist of the core and the shell (see Figure 7.7). Physical trappings, covalent bonding or electrostatic force can be used to incorporate the desired pharmaceuticals. Micellar nanoparticles incorporating doxorubicin (Matsumura *et al.*, 2004) and paclitaxel (Hamaguchi *et al.*, 2005) are currently undergoing clinical study in Japan. When they are intravenously injected, they can avoid the reticuloendothelial system (RES) and are therefore able to circulate for a long time in the bloodstream and accumulate in cancer tissues via the enhanced permeation and retention (EPR) effect. To date, the clinical data look promising, with the products under development exhibiting fewer side-effects than their conventional counterparts.

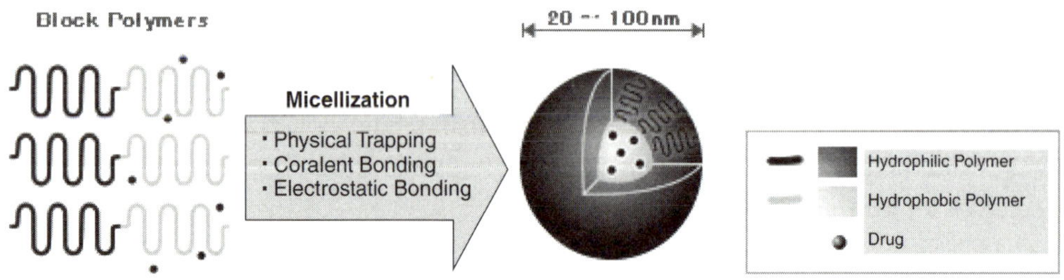

Reproduced by kind permission of NanoCarrier Co. Ltd.

Figure 7.7 Polymer micelle drug

6. Examples are: NanoCrystal™ (Elan Corporation, plc); NANOEDGE ™ (Baxter Healthcare Corporation); and Biorise™ (Eurand)

COMPLIANCE-RELATED PACKAGING

Solid dosage forms

Press-through pack (PTP) or blisters

With respect to PTP blisters, there are two issues relating to compliance. The first concerns the materials used. Japanese patients and medical staff prefer to use transparent sheets, which allow the easy identification of the dosage forms packed inside. Thus blisters composed of aluminium sheets are quite rare. There is also the issue of handling moisture-sensitive products when blistered. In Japan, tablets are initially blistered with transparent films using aluminium sheet backings, and then the blistered sheets are packed into an aluminium pouch with a desiccant. The stability of the product in this final packaging is confirmed and these data are then submitted for a New Drug Application (NDA).[7]

Stability studies of products in blisters themselves, after removal from an aluminium pouch, are also conducted, and relevant information is provided to the dispensing pharmacists as interview forms. Polyvinyl chloride (PVC) and polyvinylidine chloride (PVDC) have been commonly used to make the transparent films for blister packaging. However, they both contain chloride, which is a potential source of dioxin when burned. Now many pharmaceutical companies in Japan are using polypropylene (PP) film as an alternative. In addition, PP film is considered to be a better barrier against moisture than PVC and almost equivalent in effectiveness to PVDC.

In the past, PTP blisters often had slits placed in them in order to make it easier for patients to tear off and separate each tablets or capsules. Unfortunately there were cases where patients attempted to use the product without removing them from the packaging, resulting in severe injuries to the throat. In view of these incidents, pharmaceutical companies in Japan have now changed their strategy and only provide horizontal slits for the PTP blisters (see Figure 7.8), which means that even if a patient tears off part of the packaging it will contain two or more units of dosage forms (Kuroyama *et al.*, 2002). Since this approach has been employed, thankfully there have been no recorded instances of the accidental swallowing of PTP pieces.

Desiccants and oxygen adsorbents

Many pharmaceuticals tend to be sensitive to heat, light, moisture and oxygen. One of the biggest problems for manufacturers is protecting pharmaceuticals from heat. As long-term stability data are collected by storing products at 25°C and 60 per cent relative humidity in order to characterize shelf life at room temperature, it is extremely important to note that, in Japan, room temperature is defined as being between 1°C and 30°C, whereas in the USA it is defined as being between 15°C and 30°C and in Europe as between 15°C and 25°C.

To protect APIs from moisture, they are packed in tight containers with or without desiccants. To avoid the effects of light, products are frequently packed in a paper box or PTP blisters with light shielding film.

7. New Drug Application: regulatory process underpinning drug approval.

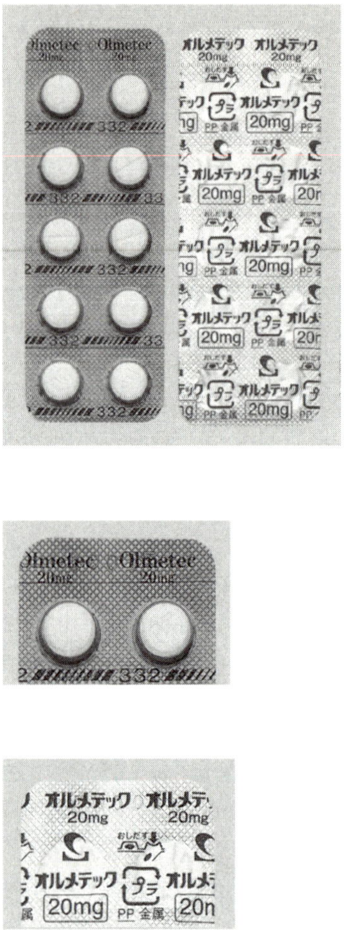

Reproduced by kind permission of Sankyo Co. Ltd.

Figure 7.8 PTB blisters with horizontal slits

To protect them from oxygen, an oxygen adsorbent – for example, Ageless®[8] the main component of which is powdered iron – is commonly used to adsorb oxygen from the atmosphere. An oxygen concentration of less than 0.1 per cent can be achieved using this measure.

Injections

Labels

Once an injectable medicine has been reconstituted within an ampoule or a vial and then transferred to a syringe or mixed with an infusion, it can be difficult to remember or write its name on the syringe or on the infusion bag from which the drugs are dispensed. This increases the potential risk of medical mistakes. Recently some vials and ampoules have

8. Manufactured by Mitsubishi Gas Chemical Co. Ltd.

been developed possessing tear-off attachable labels (see Figure 7.9), which are then pasted on to the syringe or the bag (Noda, 2003). This minimizes potential medical mistakes, which consequently improves patients' confidence and enhances compliance.

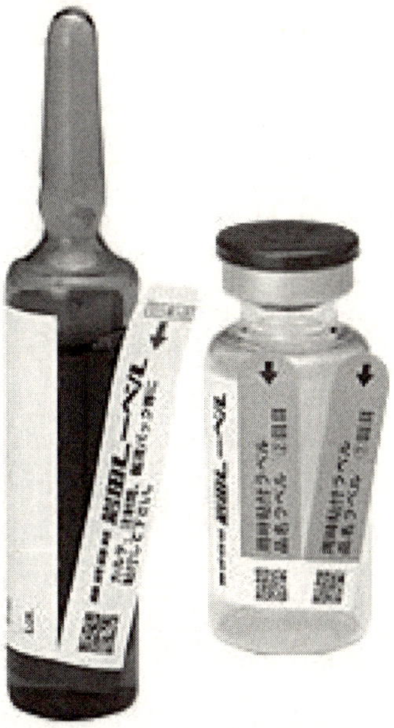

Reproduced by kind permission of Iwata Label Co., Ltd

Figure 7.9 Tear-off attachable labels

The application of oxygen adsorbent to parenterals

Sodium bisulphite is formulated for some parenteral products, such as amino acid infusions filled in ampoules or vials, in order to stabilize them from oxidation by reducing the dissolved oxygen level, and atmospheric substitution with nitrogen gas. A number of infusion products packaged in soft bags have been recently manufactured, but because air can easily penetrate the bags, additional methods of reducing oxygen levels are required. One alternative way of protecting the products from oxidation involves using nitrogen gas substitution and oxygen adsorbents, mentioned earlier. Oxygen adsorbents are inserted when the infusion bags are placed and sealed in gas barrier films. In this way, sodium bisulphite can be excluded from the formulation, which avoids excessive exposure to this compound; this is naturally considered better for patients, particularly as infusions are classified as large-volume parenterals.

Additional forms of packaging for compliance

A variety of measures to improve patients' compliance with solid and parenteral dosage forms have been discussed above. Below, some additional measures, currently being discussed in Japan, are reported.

Athlete's foot medication and eye drops

Containers for tinctures for athlete's foot and those for eye drops sometimes cause confusion amongst Japanese patients. There have been instances in Japan where patients have mistaken one product for the other. To prevent this medical mistake, the Federation of Pharmaceutical Manufacturers' Association of Japan has examined a number of potential countermeasures. It has been suggested that the products could be differentiated in terms of:

1. filling volume: in Japan the abbreviations 'NLT' 10ml for athlete's foot and 'NMT' 5ml for eye drops could be used
2. using different nozzle colours
3. using different mechanisms for application, such as a push-out or spray for athlete's foot products.

Thrombin products

In Japan, thrombin solution is often applied to stop topical bleeding. This used to be marketed in a glass vial in order to give the impression of quality. Although the sign 'Do not inject' was clearly marked on the label, there were a number of instances where the product was accidentally injected. To avoid this problem the container has now been changed from a glass vial to a soft bottle, as shown in Figure 7.10 (*Nikkan Kogyo Shimbun*, 2005).

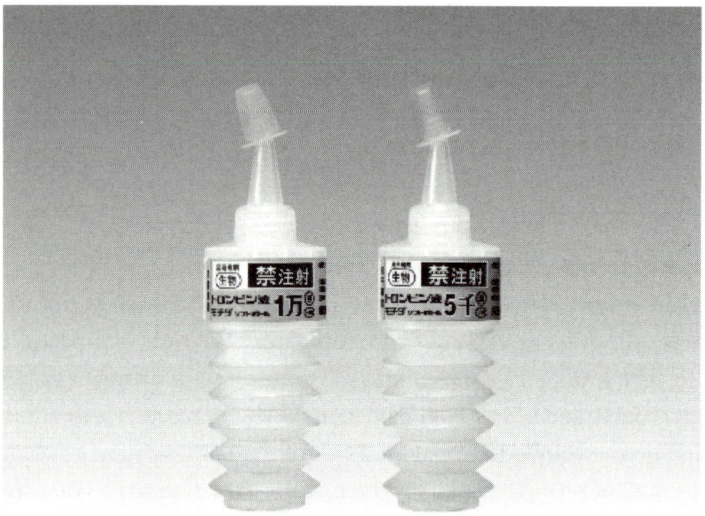

Figure 7.10 Soft bottles with bellows

COMPLIANCE IN RELATION TO DISPENSING COUNTERS

Solid dosage forms

Grinding tablets at the dispensing counter

In Japan, it is common for dispensing pharmacists to grind tablets into powders to assist patients who have difficulties when swallowing tablets. To support Japanese pharmacists in this regard, pharmaceutical companies are expected to provide them with information on the stability of tablets after the grinding process, even though the companies may not have intended their products to be ground up. For example, a *Handbook on the Milling of Tablets and Capsules* (Sagawa and Mizoguchi, 2003) is now available in Japan. The data contained in this publication were supplied by all the major Japanese pharmaceutical companies. This is important given that, once subjected to grinding, the product's stability against light and moisture will be inferior to that of the original tablets. Furthermore, the ground product may change in taste and smell and adhesions to the mortar or tools used to prepare the ground product can prevent accurate dosing. This aspect of the Japanese pharmaceutical market must be considered, as there are several machines suitable for grinding available to pharmacists at dispensing counters (see Figure 7.11 for an example). Although perhaps obvious, it should be noted that tablets such as controlled-release tablets are not suitable for grinding at such outlets.

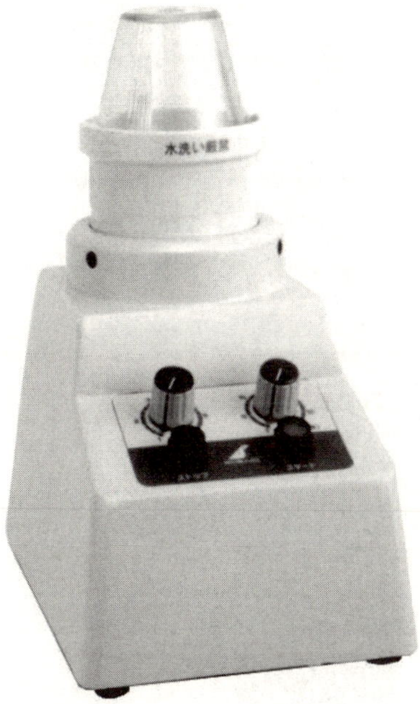

Figure 7.11 Tablet milling machine

Currently, an easy suspension method is employed as an alternative means of solving the swallowing problems commonly seen in elderly patients. This involves placing a tablet or a capsule in a syringe, pouring 20 ml of water at a temperature of 55°C and allowing this to stand for up to 10 minutes (Kurata, 2002).

Unit-dose pack

Sometimes, several types of drug are prescribed for patients, especially for those who suffer from chronic diseases. However, the dosing interval may be different from drug to drug – some may be administered three times daily, some twice daily, whilst others may only be administered once daily.

To support patients in their need to take the correct dose of each medication at the right time, unit-dose packing is commonly employed by dispensing pharmacies. Each sachet contains all the drugs that are expected to be administered at any given time. Fully automatic machines for preparing unit-dose packs are now on the market in Japan[9] and have greatly assisted pharmacists in ensuring the proper administration of products to patients (see Figure 7.12).

Furthermore, the actual preparation of these unit-dose packs is considered to be an integral skill of pharmacists, and so they can charge patients for this service. When the pharmaceuticals are placed in the cassettes of the dispensing machine, they are unpackaged. To guarantee that the product retains its quality even when used in the machine, pharmaceutical companies in Japan provide stability data for tablets and capsules without any packaging (Japanese Society of Hospital Pharmacists, 2003).

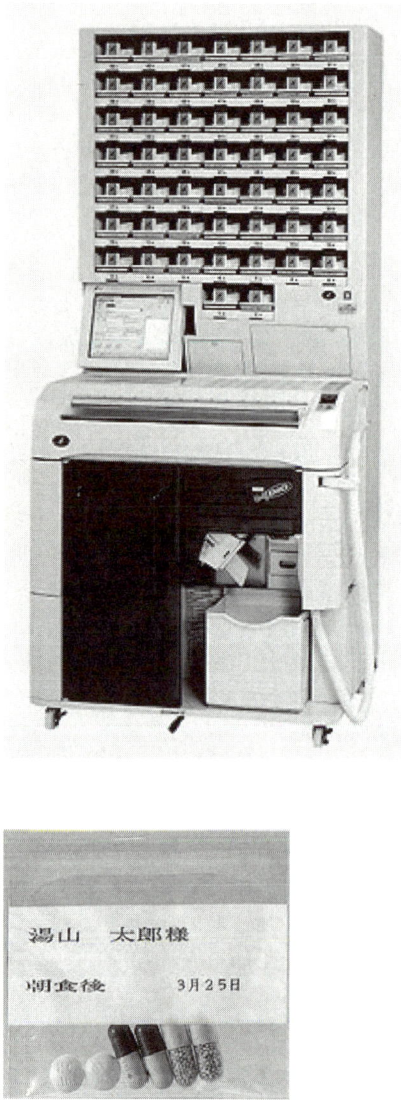

Reproduced by kind permission of Takazono Sangyo Co. Ltd and Yuyama Co. Ltd.

Figure 7.12 A fully automatic machine for unit-dose packing

---

9. Manufactured by companies such as Takazono Sangyo Co. Ltd, Yuyama Co., DAIDOKAKO Co. Ltd, and Konishi.

Half-tablets

Break lines for tablets have been introduced in Japan to allow the dose for a drug to be adjusted. Dispensing counters are often short of space and so pharmacists are limited in how many shelves they can use for drugs. This means that making the best use of this space is an important consideration for Japanese pharmacists, although this is something that is often overlooked by outside observers. It is in this regard that using break lines for drugs finds favour with pharmacists. For example, with drugs that are marketed in different doses, the pharmacist may stock the higher-strength version but still be able to provide a patient with lower dose by breaking the tablet in two.

Patients who are to create half-tablets for themselves are asked to divide tablets manually or with a knife. They are advised to apply pressure to the tablet on the opposite side to the break line using the convex side of a spoon. As an alternative, specialized tablet cutters or pill cutters are sold in the USA and can be ordered over the Internet.

However, when half-tablets are dispensed in Japan, they are usually divided and dispensed at the dispensing counter. This is done by special automatic and semi-automatic tablet-breaking tools that are marketed in Japan (see Figure 7.13). Again, dispensing pharmacists are able to charge for the service of dividing tablets in this manner.

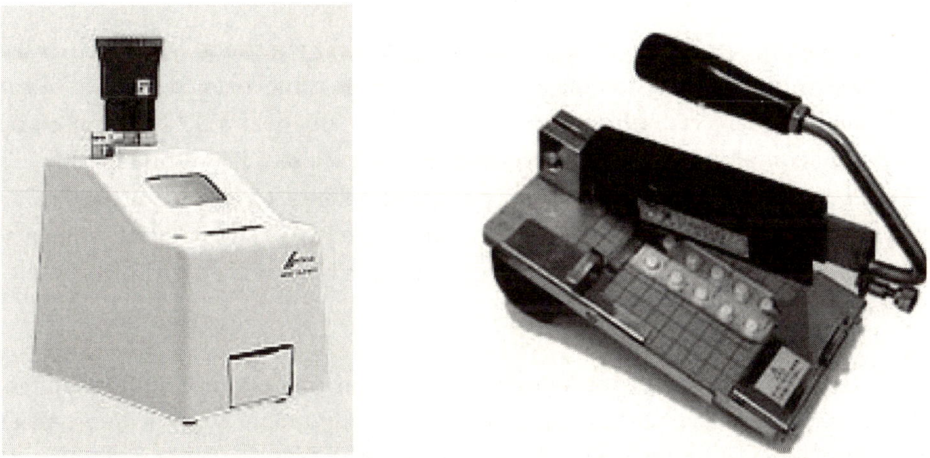

Reproduced by kind permission of Takazono Sangyo Co. Ltd and Daido Kako Co. Ltd.

Figure 7.13 Tools for preparing half-tablets

CONCLUSION: FORMULATING FOR COMPLIANCE

This chapter has attempted to provide an insight into the myriad factors that have a bearing on patient compliance in Japan. Some factors are familiar to an international audience and are analogous to medical practice in their home markets. However, other compliance factors have their origins in the style of medical treatment that was offered in the past, particularly with respect to Chinese herbal medicines, and relate to traditional Japanese cultural attitudes.

As has been discussed, the role of the Japanese pharmacist will also have an impact on the types of medicine that are made available to patients in the future. It will be important to gain the confidence of these healthcare personnel if new therapies are to be successful in improving compliance. Through their interactions with the public, pharmacists have practical experience of what is considered acceptable by Japanese patients and understand which factors affect their attitudes towards a product. Companies are recognizing the role of the pharmacist and, when necessary, have provided them with additional data on their products to facilitate dispensing.

Modern Japan is an industrialized society and because of this there is a keen interest in novel technologies. The range of technologies being applied to daily life in Japan suggests that patients will welcome their application to medicine. As has been discussed in this chapter, pharmaceutical scientists and others involved in product development are exploring a range of technologies to determine how they can make pharmaceuticals more patient-friendly and gain a patient's confidence in using a medicine. In some cases, reducing medical errors through new product development approaches has proved a useful means of improving patient compliance.

One technology area that is advancing rapidly is that for injections. Most patients dislike injections, but the nature of some of the candidate molecules being developed restricts their delivery to injectable forms, so developments in this field will have a major bearing on patient compliance. Diabetes serves as one clear example. The World Health Organization has estimated that the prevalence of diabetes in Japan was around 6.7 million in 2000 but will increase to nearly 9 million by 2030 (WHO, 2005). Since many patients currently have to endure insulin injections, advances in this field will be welcomed.

Japan is a major world pharmaceutical market, and pharmaceutical consumption remains high. Given the rate at which Japanese society is ageing and the types of disease that tend to affect this section of the population, the demand for medicines is set to increase. Only by addressing compliance issues can companies ensure that the medicines they develop meet the expectations of Japanese patients and gain their favour.

REFERENCES

Akiyama, Y. (2001), 'Adhesive Micromatrix System (AdMMS), as an Oral Sustained-Release Drug Delivery System and as a Targeting Drug Delivery System to Gastrointestinal Tract', *Pharm Tech Japan*, **17**, pp. 905–21.

Akiyama, Y., Yoshioka, Y., Horibe, H., Hirai, S., Kitamori, N. and Toguchi, H. (1993), 'Nobel Oral Controlled–release Microspheres using Polyglycerol Esters of Fatty Acids', *Journal of Controlled Release*, **26**, pp. 1–10.

Ansell, J. (2005), 'Growth Areas for Fixed Combinations', 18th Interfex Japan, Tokyo, May.

Asakura, T. and Seino, H. (2004), 'Basic Study on a Micro-tapered Needle (TN-3305) Used for Insulin Pre-filled Products', *Japanese Journal of Pharmacological Health Care Science*, **30**(6), pp. 368–76.
Asahi Shimbun (2005), 22 January.
Benameur, H. (2003), 'Formulation of Poorly Soluble Actives: How to Make it an Industrial Reality', Capsugel Symposium on Oral Delivery of Poorly Soluble Actives – From Drug Discovery to Marketed Products, Tokyo, June.
Drug Approval and Licensing Procedures in Japan 1998 (1999), Tokyo: Yakugyo Jiho.
Hamaguchi, T., Matsumura, Y., Suzuki, M., Shimizu, K., Goda, R., Nakamura, I., Nakatomi, I., Yokoyama, M., Kataoka, K. and Kakizoe, T. (2005), 'NK105, a Paclitaxel-incorporating Miceller Nanoparticle Formulation, Can Extend in Vivo Antitumor Activity and Reduce the Neuro Toxicity of Paclitaxel', *British Journal of Cancer*, **92**, pp. 1240–46.
Hata, T., Shimazaki, Y., Kagayama, A., Tamura, S. and Ueda, S. (1994), 'Development of a Novel Drug Delivery System, Time-controlled Explosion System (TES): V. Animal Pharmacodynamic Study and Human Bioavailability Study', *International Journal of Pharmacology*, **110**, pp. 1–7.
Hirayama, T., Kuroyama, M., Yago, K. and Shimada, S. (1999), 'Usefulness of Kit Products for Injection – The Usefulness of a Powder-and-Diluent Kit Packed in a Non-glass Container', *Pharm Tech Japan*, **15**(7), pp. 1065–72.
Hoshi, N., Ogura, T., Shimamoto. T. and Uramatsu, S. (2003), 'Development of PVA Copolymer Capsules', *Pharm Tech Japan*, **19**(1), pp. 17–30.
Ishino, R., Yoshino, H., Hirakawa, Y. and Noda, K. (1992), 'Design and Preparation of Pulsatile Release Tablet as a New Oral Drug Delivery System', *Chemical and Pharmaceutical Bulletin*, **40**(11), pp. 3036–41.
Izumi, M. (1999), 'The Agenda for the Development of Dual Chamber Plastic Bag Kit – Parenteral Powder Drug (Dry Drug) and Diluent', *Pharm Tech Japan*, **15**(9), pp. 1383–89.
Japanese Society of Hospital Pharmacists (ed.) (2003), *Information on the Stability of Tablets and Capsules without Packaging*, Tokyo: Iyaku (Medical and Drug) Journal Co. Ltd.
Kataoka, K. (2000), 'Nanoparticle Formulation from Polymeric Micelles', *Pharm Tech Japan*, **16**(8), pp. 1209–19.
Kawashima, Y. (2004), 'Biodegradable Polymeric Nanoparticulate System for DDS', *Pharm Tech Japan*, **20**, pp. 25–40.
Kurata, N. (2002), 'Medication Support to a Patient with a Handicap – New Method of Administration in Tube Feeding – Simple Suspension Method', *Pharm Tech Japan*, **19**(3), pp. 435–41.
Kuroyama, M., Hirayama, T., Yago, K. and Shimada, S. (1999a), 'Usefulness of Kit Products for Injection', *Pharm Tech Japan*, **15**(7), pp. 1065–72.
Kuroyama, M., Hirayama, T., Yago, K. and Shimada, S. (1999b), 'Usefulness of Prefilled Syringe Kit', *Pharm Tech Japan*, **15**(12), pp. 1865–70.
Kuroyama, M., Matsumoto, K. and Yago, K. (2002), 'Mistaken Ingestion of Tablet/Capsule PTP (Press Through Packages) and Preventive Measures', *Pharm Tech Japan*, **18**(5), pp. 769–73.
Liversidge, G. (2002), 'Abstract of the 12th Meeting of the Japan Society of Pharmaceutical Machinery and Engineering', Tokyo, October.
Liversidge, G. (2004), 'Abstract of the 2nd Symposium on Pharmaceutical Technology', Tokyo, July.

Matsumura, Y., Hamaguchi, T., Ura, T., Muro, K., Yamada, Y., Shirao, K., Okusaka, T., Ueno, H., Ikeda, M. and Watanabe, N. (2004), 'Phase I Clinical Trial and Pharmacokinetic Evaluation on NK911, Amiceller Incorporated Doxorubicin', *British Journal of Cancer*, **91**, pp. 1775–81.

Morishita, M. (2002), 'Recent Trend of Transmucosal Insulin Delivery System', *Pharm Tech Japan*, **18**(12), pp. 2077–82.

Nagai, N. (editorial supervisor), Compatibility Study on Injections Team at Koseinenkin Hospital (ed.) (1999), *Useful Handbook at Ward on Compatibility of Injections*, Tokyo: Iyaku (Medical and Drug) Journal Co. Ltd.

Nagata S. (2004), 'Drug Product in Japan', in M. Hashida (ed.), 'Future Prospect of Pharmaceutical Development and Technology 2004', *Pharm Tech Japan*, **20**(4), pp. 611–615.

Narisawa, S., Nagata, M., Danyoshi, C., Yoshino, H., Murata, K., Hirakawa, Y. and Noda, K. (1994), 'An Organic Acid-Induced Sigmoidal Release System for Oral Controlled-Release Preparations', *Pharmaceutical Research*, **11**(1), pp. 111–16.

Nikkan Kogyo Shimbun (2005), 6 January.

Nikkei Sangyo Shimbun (2005), 25 May.

Nishioka, J., Komoike, J., Tozaki, H., Yamamoto, A., Muranishi, S., Kim, S.I. and Terashima, H. (1997), 'Colon Delivery of Physiological Active Peptide with Azopolymer-Coated Pellets', Abstract of the Japanese Society for the Study of Xenobiotics 12th Annual Meeting.

Noda, K. (2003), 'How Does the Packaging Maker Wrestle against the Medication Error?', *Gekkan Yakuji*, **45**(11), pp. 2001–2005.

Ogura, T., Ohsuga, K., Tomita, K., Furuya, Y. and Takagishi, Y. (1998), 'New Cellulose Capsules', *Pharm Tech Japan*, **14**(3), pp. 391–400.

Okada, H. (1997), 'One-and Three-month Release Injectable Microspheres of the LH-RH Superagonist Leuprorelin Acetate', *Advanced Drug Delivery Reviews*, **28**, pp. 43–70.

Okada, H. (1998), 'Dosage and Design of Leuprorelin Acetate Microspheres for Long-term Sustained-release Injection', *Pharm Tech Japan*, **14**(1), pp. 75–88.

Okada, K. (1999), 'Guidance to Raw Materials used for Gelatin Production in Europe and the US', *Pharm Tech Japan*, **15**(5), pp. 671–74.

Onuki, H. (2004), 'Proposal of Nobel Capsules', *Pharm Tech Japan*, **20**(2), pp. 308–309.

Onuki, Y. and Okabe, H. (2004), 'Design and Characteristics of Patches for Transdermal Therapeutic Systems', *Pharm Tech Japan*, **20**(5), pp. 979–84.

Otsuka, T. (2001), 'Safety Assurance of Gelatin Concerning BSE', *Pharm Tech Japan*, **17**(9), pp. 1407–11.

Pharmacopoeia of Japan (2001), Vol. XIV at: http://jpdb.nihs.go.jp/jp14e.

Rabinow, B.E. (2004), 'Nanosuspension in Drug Delivery', *Pharm Tech Japan*, **20**(12), pp. 2357–76.

Sagawa, K. and Mizoguchi, K. (eds) (2003), *Handbook on the Milling of Tablets and Capsules*, Tokyo: Jiho Co.

Sako, K. (1998) 'Design of Novel Oral Controlled-Release System (OCAS) for Continuous Drug Absorption', *Pharm Tech Japan*, **14**(6), pp. 869–82.

Sako, K., Nakashima, H., Sawada, T. and Fukui, M. (1996), 'Relationship between Gelation Rate of Controlled-release Acetaminophen Tablets Containing Polyethylene Oxide and Colonic Drug Release in Dogs', *Pharmaceutical Research*, **13**, pp. 594–98.

Sano, A., Hojo, T., Maeda, M. and Fujioka, K. (1998), 'Protein Release from Collagen Matrices', *Advanced Drug Delivery Reviews*, **31**(3), pp. 247–66.

Sano, A., Maeda, M., Nagahara, S., Ochiya, T., Honma, K., Itoh, H., Miyata, T. and Fujioka, K. (2003), 'Atelocollagen for Protein and Gene Delivery', *Advanced Drug Delivery Reviews*, **55**(12), pp. 1651–77.

Seta, Y., Otsuka, T., Tokiwa, H., Naganuma, H., Kawahara, Y., Nishimura, K. and Okada, R. (1988), 'Design of Captopril Sustained-release Preparation with Oily Semisolid Matrix Intended for Use in Human Subjects', *International Journal of Pharmacology*, **41**, pp. 263–69.

Sugihara, M. (1994), 'Novel Dosage Forms and Packaging Suitable for Elderly Patients', *Farumasia*, **30**(12), pp. 1396–400.

Takahasi, Y., Ishihara T. and Kashihara, T. (1998),'Current Status on Selection of Excipients in Japanese Pharmaceutical Companies', in M. Hshida (ed.), *Formulation Design of Oral Dosage Forms*, Tokyo: Yakugyojiho, pp. 120–37.

Todo, H., Ishida, K., Okamoto, H. and Danjo, K. (2002), 'Efficacy and Safety of Insulin Dry Powders for Inhalation', *Pharm Tech Japan*, **18(**1), pp. 83–93.

Tsushima, Y. (2004), 'Current Trend on User-friendly Dosage Forms', *Farumashia*, **40**(9), pp. 817–21.

WHO (2005), 'Diabetes Programme', at: http://www.who.int/diabetes/en/.

CHAPTER 8

Sweetening the Pill: Compliance and Clinical Trials

Dr Graham Wylie, Mike Bradburn, Dr Brian Edwards, Tanwen Evans and Dr Richard Kay

Compliance is important. Better adherence to treatment regimes leads to less healthcare resource utilization overall, as fewer illness recurrence or medication errors leading to side-effects take place. Traditionally, we have seen a conflict between assessments of the efficacy of treatments and the assessment of effectiveness of treatments. Some trials are designed to test the maximal effect of a treatment (that is, efficacy), which others argue is unrealistic and therefore misleading. This group argues for trials based on 'real-world' scenarios (that is, effectiveness). This conflict is natural and inevitable as both objectives are valid, assuming that the trial environment can be replicated in a meaningful way in routine medical care. Furthermore, the conflict can be minimized by accepting that both objectives can be assessed in a competent development plan for a new treatment, answering all critical questions.

We have split the issues of compliance and clinical trials into two categories – compliance as a variable in the study to be managed and compliance as the primary endpoint to be studied. Within this discussion, compliance will be defined as the level of adherence to treatment regimes. We touch on the issue of population effects by outlining some of the related methods of ensuring correct prescribing in the first place; these increase the level of treatment reaching the population as a whole, not just an individual patient. Statistical treatment of compliance is covered, showing how a thoughtful and sophisticated approach gives us more information about both key objectives of efficacy and effectiveness, and outlines some rarely used modelling techniques that address the issue.

Lastly, we will look at the trials that treat compliance as an endpoint in itself. These are usually post marketing trials, sponsored either by academics within the healthcare system or by pharmaceutical companies. It is often assumed that these different sponsors treat the subject quite differently, leading to some heated debate over the quality of the research. In my view, most of the work is actually quite compatible, and indeed very similar, albeit approached from different perspectives. It is important to see past such simplistic views and assess the research for its true worth – regardless of sponsor. When this is done, good work is produced by both sponsor groups, adding to our overall knowledge of healthcare delivery. Both groups' data point to the fact that a more interactive process of healthcare delivery increases the effectiveness of treatments.

Our overall conclusion is that the majority of research indicates that, for many conditions (but probably not all), a paradigm shift is needed away from our centralized system to a distributed, home-based delivery of care and treatment, with appropriate disintermediation (that is, automation) to reduce costs where possible. This is because our traditional approach of heavily centralized healthcare only touches patients at infrequent intervals, usually at clinic visits, whereas patients have to cope with their condition every day, in their normal work and leisure routine and environment. It is overcoming this barrier that is fundamentally addressed by all methods of increasing compliance – either by using electronic tools or, for example, through healthcare delivered at home. If increasing compliance reduces costs and improves health, then the paradigm must change.

WHY IS COMPLIANCE IMPORTANT?

The best way of answering this question is to look at the objectives of the stakeholders – stakeholders being the producers, the buyers, the regulators, the prescribers and the patients. Essentially all the stakeholders will want the same things:

- They want to study drug effects cost-effectively and want to have the best chance of demonstrating overall benefit to patients.
- They want the best health impact for the cost of the product.
- They want drugs that will work in the real world, within a meaningful (by which is normally meant 'large') patient population.

These driving forces can be in conflict, so they need to be in an overall balance. In practice this usually means achieving a balance between the desires and needs of the science versus the practical application of the treatment in the real world – or, simply put, 'efficacy versus effectiveness'. Neither of these approaches is right or wrong; they are simply forces that need to be considered by all stakeholders, none of whom have a vested interest in losing the balance. Having said that, we do believe in general that all stakeholders have an interest in achieving *high* compliance, *as long as* what is studied in trials can be translated to the real world at a later stage.

The following two sections deal with this issue of efficacy versus effectiveness from somewhat different perspectives. The first section – compliance as a variable – has a research and development (R&D) perspective, and covers the factors that govern compliance behaviour in clinical trials, tools to improve compliance and the best statistical treatment of the data to demonstrate both efficacy and effectiveness. The second section – compliance as an endpoint – has a more commercial and 'real-world' perspective, and covers the assessment of compliance as a key outcome where the boundaries between studies and routine medical care start to blur. The chapter finishes with an analysis of the lessons which cross over from the trial environment to routine medical practice and a summary of the main points of the chapter as a whole.

COMPLIANCE AS A VARIABLE

In a clinical trial comparing treatments, compliance plays a key role in determining the effect of the therapy and is treated as a variable which should be controlled between the comparative groups. This means that the hypothesis being tested for superiority, equivalence or non-inferiority will rely on the two treatment groups showing similar patterns of compliance. Whilst this is fine for other variables which are not clearly linked to outcome – perhaps the distribution of the males and females between the groups – for compliance this approach is somewhat risky as a lack of compliance may be directly related to the efficacy and safety objectives of the study. In other words, groups may look the same in an analysis because patients who experience side-effects or a lack of efficacy tend to drop out or fail to take their medication. Where treatment groups have different compliance behaviours, this makes interpretation of the key objectives of the study difficult. The 'intent-to-treat' analysis will control for this effect but tends to underestimate the overall efficacy of the treatment. To manage this risk to the clarity of the results, compliance should be carefully measured in all treatment groups, preferably in several ways, and efforts should be made to achieve the highest compliance rates possible so that the underlying effects of the treatments can be determined. Of course, this creates trials which are less like 'real life' than we would hope, creating the efficacy versus effectiveness conundrum. Scientifically, the best way of tackling this is initially to carry out studies focused on the possible effect of the treatment, followed by studies that are closer to real-life therapy situations, which can then differentiate between the potential effect of the treatment and the actual effect, taking compliance into account. This progression of objectives through a development programme of this sort allows complex interactions to be teased apart. Of course, we not only want to know what happens within a population of patients to see if the treatments are effective overall, but also what is the expected benefit for individual patients who do comply with therapy; both are identified by this overall approach.

Enhancing compliance

Research on factors affecting adherence or compliance in clinical trials has been scarce, with few investigations to evaluate strategies for enhancing patient participation. One reason may be the absence of a conceptual framework to guide research. Many opinions about why patients do not comply have been extrapolated from experience and observations in normal clinical use. Non-compliance in clinical trials is believed to be much lower because of volunteers' willingness to participate in research although, naturally, this hypothesis is difficult to confirm, as the circumstances in interventionist studies are so different.

As a rule, patients cannot be simply classified as compliers or non-compliers. Rather, the level of compliance ranges from patients who take every prescribed dose precisely as directed to those who never do with the typical patient lying between these two extremes. The degree to which patients intend to comply with a regimen can be subdivided into patient-controlled and structural. Patient-controlled factors can be subdivided further into rational behaviour (as seen in patients with Parkinson's disease who regulate their own dosing) and irrational behaviours (such as self-induced seizures). Structural factors are those beyond the patient's control, such as impaired memory or difficulty accessing medication (Leppik, 1990).

Patients who deceive

There are always some patients who admit that they do not take the treatment as prescribed. However, some patients may deliberately deceive doctors. Indeed, the patients who deceive doctors are often the individuals one least suspects. A good example is treatment for asthma since technology is available to assess compliance – for example, the Nebuliser Chronolog™. In a study of 19 patients studied for 12 weeks, using such technology, appropriate usage four times a day ranged from 4.3 per cent to 94.8 per cent. Underusage exceeded overusage and ranged from 5.2 per cent to 95 per cent of the study days. Patients failed to write the truth in their diaries, over-reporting appropriate usage more than 50 per cent of the time (Spector *et al.*, 1986).

In a five-year follow-up study of 101 patients with chronic obstructive pulmonary disease (COPD), 30 patients activated their inhalers more than 100 times within a three-hour interval on at least one occasion during the first year of follow-up. Most of these dumping episodes occurred shortly before a clinic follow-up, suggesting that patients were actively attempting to hide non-compliance from clinic staff (Simmons *et al.*, 2000). Although, in this trial, no predictors of dumping could be found, trial participants with dumping behaviour are otherwise ideal research subjects. They get on well with staff. They can be relied on to complete questionnaires and show up for follow-up clinic visits. In other words, they are the very patients who do not want to disappoint their physician.

Factors behind non-compliance

Compliance depends on many factors, including the study population (better in educated compared to disadvantaged patients) type of intervention, duration of treatment, complexity of treatment, real or perceived side-effects and life circumstances (see Table 8.1). The reasons are often patient-specific, multifaceted and can change over time. Demographically, the very young, the very old, teenagers and those taking very complex treatment regimes are the least likely to comply. Common examples of adverse reactions affecting compliance are those affecting the central nervous system (such as sedation and dizziness) and cosmetic events (such as hirsutism and weight gain). Larger studies have found no worthwhile or significant difference in levels of compliance between once- and twice-daily regimens. However three-, four- or more times daily regimens involving more than four drugs are difficult to take correctly (Greenberg, 1984; Pullar *et al.*, 1988; Taggart *et al.*, 1981; Farup, 1992).

Table 8.1 Factors affecting patient compliance

Limited access to medications	• Inability to drive or transportation difficulty • No time to obtain medication
Increased complexity of dosing regimen	• Inconvenient, frequent or complicated dosing schedule • Polytherapy • Misunderstanding, anxiety or confusion over dosing schedule
Poor education	• Difficulty understanding how to use the medication, the nature of disease being treated and the reason for treatment
Medical factors	• Adverse reactions to the medication • Cognitive or neurological effects of the disease itself • Other co-morbid conditions
Psychosocial factors	• Weak support from family and friends • Poor relationship with the investigator or own referring physician • Fear of adverse effects • Denial of disease • Financial or other problems in coping with life • Feeling better and so developing a lax attitude, or discontinuing to see if cured

The author of a literature review based on about 12 000 publications (half of them review articles and half reporting original data) has suggested that good compliance is related to:

- patients' satisfaction
- continuity of care, and
- acceptance of the need for treatment.

Poor (patient-controlled) compliance was associated with:

- chronic, asymptomatic disorders
- complex treatment regimens
- adverse effects, and
- social dysfunction (Blackwell, 1996).

In a publication 20 years earlier, the same author identified that asymptomatic and chronic diseases needing long-term treatment, such as depressive illnesses, result in poorer compliance; and that the longer the remission in chronic diseases, the lower the compliance (Blackwell, 1976). Finally, another publication showed that patient-controlled non-compliance was lower in treatment for diseases in which the relationship between non-compliance and recurrence is very clear, such as diabetes, compared to treatment for diseases in which this relationship is less clear, such as depressive disorder (Kirscht and Rosenstock, 1980). Of course, cognitive deficit, helplessness, poor motivation and withdrawal all lead to forgetfulness and passive or structural non-compliance (Gitlin *et al.*, 1989; Shaw, 1986).

Differences between compliance in observational and interventionist studies

How representative are compliance data from observational studies compared to interventionist studies? In the case of anti-depressants, average discontinuation rates are lower in observational studies, suggesting that compliance is higher in interventionist trials than in normal clinical practice. In turn, this suggests that risk factors for non-compliance from clinical trials are not the same as those for non-compliance in clinical practice. Furthermore, discontinuation rates are significantly higher in placebo-controlled, three-arm studies compared to two-arm comparative studies (for example, about 20–25 per cent in depression studies with selective serotonin reuptake inhibitors (SSRIs)). This suggests that the less the investigator knows about who is getting the active product (compared to a placebo), the higher will be the discontinuation rate. However, the way in which discontinuation rates are reported differs between observational and interventionist studies, as may the rigour of follow-up. In general, the reasons recorded are often rather broad: 'death'; 'due to side-effects', 'due to lack of efficacy' and 'others' (which can cover administrative problems, lost cases or protocol violations). Details are usually in the discontinuation narrative, if this exists. The time course of the discontinuation is important: early drop-outs are mainly due to lack of efficacy and side-effects whereas later drop–outs, beyond 12 weeks, tend to be due to feeling better or other reasons (such as fear of dependence). Finally, clinical trials are short-term and hence the results on discontinuation cannot be extrapolated to long-term treatment. Variations in the type of non-compliance are found over a period of months: in the beginning, the typical reaction is to discontinue treatment; in the mid-term, patients are more casual and often forget; and in the longer term, they begin to vary the dosage (Myers and Branthwaite, 1992).

Compliance with questionnaires and diaries

Doctors often ask patients to recall recent health experiences, such as pain, fatigue and quality of life. Research has shown, however, that recall is unreliable and rife with inaccuracies and biases. Recognition of the shortcomings of recall has led to the use of diaries, which are intended to capture experiences close to the time of occurrence, thus limiting recall bias and producing more accurate data. Inclusion of the QoL (quality of life) factor in clinical trials presents a number of difficult organizational issues, and serious problems in compliance have frequently been reported. Thus, in multicentre clinical trials many of the expected QoL questionnaires fail to be successfully completed and returned, although a few groups have claimed high success rates. However, it is well recognized that if questionnaires are missing, there may be bias in the interpretation of trial results, and the estimates of treatment differences and the overall level of QoL may be inaccurate and misleading (Fayers *et al.*, 1997).

One study, which compared electronic and paper diaries, supported concerns of compliance with paper diaries. Although patients reported high compliance, actual compliance was low and hoarding was common. The excellent compliance achieved with the electronic diary indicates that low compliance was not due to this particular sample or to an overly burdensome protocol (Stone *et al.*, 2002). This whole theme is explored in much more detail by Bill Byrom and David Stein in Chapter 10.

The regulatory implications of non-compliance

There is considerable concern about the safety and economic implications of medication errors.[1] As a result, pharmaceutical manufacturers are expected to consider how compliance problems ('medication errors') in the development programme might be extrapolated to the real-life marketing phase. This is reflected in recent guidance issued by the Food and Drug Administration (FDA) about pre-marketing risk assessment.[2] Thus, if the patient misunderstands the labelling, instructions for use or has difficulty with drug delivery this may well have implications either for future labelling, education and design for post-authorization studies. These errors could be detected by either medical or clinical monitoring, and it is important to document these findings and to review them as with any other safety data, looking for signals as part of the overall benefit–risk assessment of the product. This is consistent with recommendation of good clinical practice (GCP) (ICH 3.3.8) where it states that the investigator should promptly report changes that increase the risk to subjects and/or significantly affect trial conduct. This is reflected in the EU Clinical Trial Directive in which expeditable safety issues not only include serious and unexpected adverse reactions but also any new event relating to trial conduct such as a serious adverse event associated with trial procedures which could modify trial conduct (*Detailed Guidance*, 2004). Conceivably, if patients do not understand or comply as a result of poor trial design and implementation, this could be interpreted as a significant non-compliance within a trial. Thus not only can inadequate compliance by patients compromise data integrity and quality but there could also be regulatory implications for the sponsor who fails to adequately manage such a situation.

TOOLS AND TECHNIQUES FOR MONITORING AND IMPROVING COMPLIANCE

Tools and techniques have two main objectives, with different levels of overlap between the two:

1. See http://www.nccmerp.org https://www.medmarx.com/index.jsp.
2. See http://www.fda.gov/cder/guidance/6357/fnl.htm.

- monitoring and recording
- motivating (and thus improving).

Monitoring and recording

There is a spectrum of devices and techniques available for monitoring and recording, ranging from pill boxes marked for each day through to electronic devices that record when they are opened to gain access to the medication they contain.

Motivating health professionals and patients in a study

Motivating study staff and patients at the start of a study and maintaining that motivation throughout the study is paramount to achieving high retention of, and compliance by, patients, which ultimately influences the likelihood of the trial successfully achieving its objectives. Motivating study staff leads to adherence to both the study's clinical procedures and the inclusion/exclusion criteria, as well as diligent data recording. For patients, motivation leads them to join, and subsequently to stay in, the study and adhere to the visit schedule and treatment regimen. Given that a patient's motivation to join and remain in a study is often inextricably linked to the physician's or study nurse's perceived enthusiasm towards the study, then it is not surprising that the latter can positively influence the former.

Increasing compliance through investigators and their study staff

Study staff appreciate participating in studies that are well run and are more interesting than other studies. The satisfaction of the study site staff usually correlates positively with site performance, reflected in accelerated recruitment, recruitment of the right type of patients and more accurate and timely recording of data. To achieve this, sponsors and clinical research organizations (CROs) need to ensure that their trial is managed well, so that the experience is made easy and rewarding for the investigators and their support staff. This means excellent operational management – namely:

- adhering to timelines during site qualification and initiation
- promptly resolving/responding to issues
- minimizing protocol amendments
- ensuring effective training of study staff
- supplying software technologies that work simply and correctly.

Although many of these functions are managed centrally by the sponsor or CRO, the local study monitor is often the only visible face that links the study staff to the sponsor – so this relationship must therefore be nurtured from the outset. Ultimately, trial management excellence leads to confidence and trust, respect for the trial protocol and more time for scientific dialogue.

It is also important to remember to approach the investigators and other study staff as healthcare professionals and not as subcontractors or sales targets. In order to make them feel valued and to reduce the cynicism and scepticism so often directed towards pharmaceutical companies in today's climate, investigators should be given scientific respect, should be made to feel involved in the research and should have opportunities for scientific dialogue with the study sponsor and fellow investigators. In essence, they want to feel as though they are researching something meaningful and are appreciated for their contribution to the research. It is often forgotten that, for most investigators, it is the science that gets them interested in the first place and not the free paperweight, the exotic location of the investigator meeting or the funds they will receive for their participation. Much more critical to strong motivation is being involved in the clinical research of a compound that has a novel, innovative mode of action, with the potential to provide a clinically significant advantage in terms of efficacy or safety, or considerably greater clinical effectiveness. Furthermore, if this new medication is set to enter an area of medicine in which currently effective treatments are absent or sparse, then this too is obviously a powerful incentive for trial staff and patients alike.

Key to achieving this is good communication with the investigators about the science that underlies the rationale behind the protocol. This needs to start well before the study design has all its details finalized, if only with a few key investigators who can ensure that those questions that will be meaningful to other investigators will be addressed. Although often an exercise in diplomacy and a virtuoso balancing act between the objectives of the various stakeholders, the effort is well worthwhile in the long term – not just for recruitment into the study, but also for buying-in opinion leaders to the new product's potential claim structure and the commercialization of the product once on the market. Once the designs are final and the protocol is ready for implementation, the investigator meeting presents a golden opportunity to really engage site staff in the science and the study as a whole. There is much room for improvement in the format of investigator meetings to make them more stimulating and interactive for the attendees.

Recruitment of the right type of patients into the trial by site staff requires consistent, and sometimes time-consuming, efforts to identify and recommend patients for screening. To ensure that potentially eligible patients are not missed and to minimize the time spent at this stage, providing sites with support to make this task more efficient can optimize their compliance with this important undertaking. Sites can be provided with a programme of tools that will keep the study 'top of mind' and make the scanning of every patient second nature. This is particularly important if the site is participating in several trials in parallel, some of which may be competing for the same patients. The tools may include algorithms to assist with patient case note review, eligibility cards that provide a quick reference to the inclusion/exclusion criteria, or posters, brochures and websites to reach out to patients. In addition, staff can be provided with tools, such as template letters and slide kits, to help them reach out to colleagues who may generate referrals.

A well-developed study identity (a graphics or set of graphics and an acronym name for the study) is the 'glue' that visually links all the above-mentioned tools to make them readily identifiable to the study staff. A study identity, also applied to patient materials (see below) also speaks to patients, using verbal and non-verbal languages, both of which serve to overcome barriers that might dissuade them from volunteering. Careful and thoughtful development of a creative concept that represents the graphical portion of the study identity can, through the imagery alone, convey a trial's basic values to the patient. It can convey feelings of caring and compassion, of strength and empowerment, or any other values that the patient population (or their family members, caregivers or friends) may strongly relate to and which will play a role in their decision to join the trial or not. The development of a study identity therefore requires careful research into key variables such as the patients' physical and psychological status, their geographical location, their age and societal status, their family and the role they might play in the decision.

Maintaining the motivation of patients throughout the study

Patients comply more with protocols and treatment regimes if they are motivated. Motivating patients starts with good recruitment practice – ensuring that patients have consented, are properly informed and are treated ethically, as well as being right for the study. This will be the direct outcome of the activities outlined in the section above. It is also dependent on site staff and sponsor communications providing a pleasant, encouraging and informative environment for the patients during the study.

The decision to join a clinical trial can be a difficult one for a patient. The lay community and even much of the medical community, poorly understand clinical research. The reasons for joining the trial are often (perhaps usually) poorly communicated to the patient and, frequently, the more severe the patient's condition, the worse the communication. To resolve this problem, all involved staff need to understand more about communicating to patients in this unique situation. In a communications context, the majority of patients will see entering a clinical study as a 'high-risk' decision, because they lack adequate information or have never had a similar experience for comparison. The most effective method of reducing the perception of high risk is to provide the appropriate level of information at the most appropriate time.

A common mistake made by physicians and nurses when communicating with patients about clinical research is to use low-involvement, more emotional messages which are simply expressive and don't meet patients' information needs, and therefore don't reduce the perception of high risks in making the decision to enter a clinical study. Messages to patients should stress functional attributes and benefits and be very rational in their delivery. Patients worldwide appear to have the same concerns about entering a study. They worry about:

- receiving a placebo
- being 'guinea pigs'
- obtaining access to the best treatment options.

In many healthcare systems, patients also worry about how to pay for what they need and so these patients, in particular, value the medical procedures and medications they receive at no cost in the clinical study setting.

Although obtaining patients' informed consent involves providing them with a lay summary of the trial and what their involvement will entail, it often does not strike the right chords. This is where additional support materials can bridge that communication gap. In many cases, the patients are not only faced with the decision to enter a study, but have just learnt their diagnosis or heard that their condition is worsening or changing in some way. They have to assimilate this first before approaching the trial decision. Patients want detailed information on their condition, their treatment and the study, written in a way that is easy to understand and not daunting. A wide range of materials can be produced to meet these information needs at different stages of the patient's involvement. Prior to obtaining informed consent, leaflets that give top-level information about the study or a video that can introduce the patient to the informed consent process are useful. The materials can cover issues not addressed by the lay summary included with the consent form, such as transportation, visit duration, waiting times and so on, all of which can help to make them feel more comfortable and encourage dialogue with the study staff.

The study identity is also powerful in motivating patients to enter the trial, as it sets expectations about care, information, attention, ease of access, simplicity, relevance and so on. With this in mind, it is important to design the study identity with elements specifically for the patient as well as for the site staff. The identity – as an ongoing flow of material – also serves to improve retention of the patients once enrolled. It is worth noting, however, that, if the implied promises of the trial do not materialize, the motivation to remain in the study slackens and drop-outs will occur. Thus, site staff training around a more 'customer-focused' approach to their patients is often very worthwhile. Once enrolled in the study, access to information through a website, a regular newsletter or other printed materials tailored for study patients to ensure that they continue to feel wanted and appreciated can help with retention. The materials educate and serve to communicate the study setting as a patient-friendly environment, of a clinical research situation that is accessible and useful to the patient's life, not one of test tubes, wires and impatient nurses with cold hands. In long studies in particular, a stream of communication can help them remain engaged with the study between visits.

Healthcare infrastructure

Patient compliance can also be hampered by the most unexpected reasons that are often difficult to uncover. Patients may decide to withdraw for reasons that cannot be addressed by improved education and that are unrelated to any medical issues. Many of these are related to the way in which healthcare is generally delivered – driven by history and its resultant infrastructure. Ask almost any health professional or patient for a list of common complaints about the healthcare system and you will probably get a list that includes:

- hospitals a long way from home
- difficulties with transportation and/or parking
- unpleasant buildings and waiting areas
- extended waiting times with nothing to do
- inconvenience for caregivers.

Often, patients are hesitant to raise these issues with the study nurse or their physician, so, unless there is a method in place to investigate these issues, they may go unnoticed and unresolved and cause a proportion of early and avoidable discontinuations. Specific questioning about these issues should be included in patient interviews and other types of follow-up.

Another developing approach is the provision of healthcare, both in and out of trials, at home. Given the list of concerns above and the huge impact of poor patient retention and compliance on trial budgets and accuracy, what better way to deliver trials than to provide the care at home – at least as much as possible? Of the time a patient spends in a trial, 99 per cent of it is at home. This is where they must cope with their symptoms, take their medication, change their behaviour, follow their diets and so on. A paradigm shift is needed to bring the care or trial system to the patient, rather than the other way around. This can be achieved in two main ways. The first is to use all the modern communication techniques now available to reach out to the patient at home. Intelligent use of the Internet, e-mail, short message service (SMS) text messaging, web-cams and, of course, the telephone allows the trial to touch the patient directly on a much more regular basis than just those occasions when they visit the clinic. This approach is addressed in depth in the Chapter 10 by Bill Byrom and David Stein.

The second method is to deliver the actual healthcare at home – the medication, the nurse, the equipment and even the doctor. This is obviously a complex undertaking, but the industry is already well developed outside of the trial environment. The market leader in this area, at least in the UK, is 'Healthcare at Home', which has a national delivery network based on centralized pharmacy and cold chain supply capability, as well as an army of nurses and doctors who deliver the treatment at the patient's home. When running clinical trials they operate much the same approach.

This has significant advantages. For the patient, it means all the preparation they or their carer have to make for the protocol visit is to put the kettle on! For the study staff the advantage is that they get to see the condition the study is operating within at first hand. Here they can see for themselves why compliance is good or bad – for instance, the medication is upstairs in the bathroom, and the patient cannot get up the stairs more than once a day to go to bed, or that it should be taken with food but the patient cannot cook and has no help with meals – factors that are much harder to assess from a distance. They can also do a more accurate medication count: for example, the patient will leave their tablets in their normal place and the nurse can go to get them, to see how many are really left – not infallible, but certainly an improvement. For the sponsor, not only does retention become a much more minor issue because the trial goes to the patient, but compliance also improves and is recorded more accurately. Study data are collected directly, reducing source data checking requirements, and continual patient training takes place to allow the best use of the medication. Furthermore, home delivery is probably cheaper, as the trial does not have to pay hospital overheads, transport expenses and so on. Such trials are also more automated, using technology to the full, with the result that staffing levels can be reduced as the roles of the study nurse and clinical research associate (CRA) start to merge. Although these savings are slightly offset by an increase in the number of study nurses, the overall cost should reduce.

This is an example of the lessons from real-life daily practice, which cross over into trials. Far from compliance being artificially improved in this scenario, the trial is now much more accurately reflecting the concept of disease management, where an holistic treatment regime is delivered to the patient, including not only a medicine, but also training on how to cope with their condition, advice on how to reduce the impact of symptoms, advice on coping with side-effects, encouragement to maintain their therapy for the right period of time and so on. Clearly, if compliance is an issue, then all the strategies utilized to improve it in trials need to cross over into real life, and vice versa, making this approach the one we believe needs to be watched for the future.

STATISTICAL TREATMENT OF COMPLIANCE

Routine treatment

Reporting of compliance

Randomized clinical trials published in the medical literature are effectively governed by the CONSORT statement (Moher *et al.*, 2001). This document offers no explicit guidance on how compliance should be described, aside from the following requirement:

> *Authors should report all departures from the protocol ... The nature of the protocol deviation and the exact reason for excluding participants after randomization should always be reported.*

In practice, space constraints lead to rather terse summaries of compliance, often no more than the number of patients who were deemed 'non-compliant', or sometimes merely the number of patient withdrawals. The manner in which compliance is assessed, and the degree of non-compliance leading to a protocol violation, is seldom specified. The situation is different within the pharmaceutical industry, where more details are a requirement of the regulatory reporting guidelines:

> *The measures taken to ensure and document treatment compliance should be described, e.g., drug accountability, diary cards, blood, urine or other body fluid drug level measurements, or medication event monitoring.*

The numbers of patients who were randomised, and who entered and completed each phase of the study (or each week/month of the study) should be provided, as well as the reasons for all post-randomisation discontinuations, grouped by treatment and by major reason (lost to follow-up, adverse event, poor compliance etc.).

> *Any measurements of compliance of individual patients with the treatment regimen under study and drug concentrations in body fluids should be summarised, analysed by treatment group and time interval, and tabulated.* (ICH, E3, 1995)

Industry-sponsored clinical study reports usually provide two analyses, with 'non-compliant' patients included in the primary analysis but excluded from the secondary (more details are given in the next section). To enable this, 'non-compliance' is defined by some pre-specified rule. Where the treatment is self-administered on an ongoing basis, a 'compliant' patient would (for example) take full medication on 80 per cent or more of the days in the study period, and be assessed by returned pill count and/or diary. Where therapy is administered under controlled circumstances (for example, by medically trained personnel), any non-receipt of treatment is often deemed to be non-compliance. In either case, a summary table such as that illustrated in Table 8.2 is usually presented.

Table 8.2 Shell of a typical compliance assessment table

Visit	Treatment	Control	Total
1	N (%)		
2			
3			
...			
Overall			

Analysis of data with non-compliance: the intention-to-treat (ITT) principle

Primary efficacy endpoints are generally analysed by the intention-to-treat (ITT) principle, in accordance with both CONSORT and ICH E9 (1998) guidelines. The ITT approach leads to a comparison between patients according to their assigned treatment, irrespective of compliance. Supportive (secondary) analyses are often performed on the so-called 'per protocol patient set', from which 'non-compliant' patients are excluded. The per protocol analysis has the advantage of demonstrating the expected effects that might be seen in individual patients who actually take the medication from both an efficacy and safety perspective. This 'efficacy' data is particularly useful to medical practitioners trying to decide whether to prescribe the product to an individual patient under their care. However, from a population perspective, the overall effectiveness of the product as a health investment is not as clear from the per protocol analysis. To address this question, the ICH E3 (1995) guidelines also look for consistency between these analyses:

> *Any substantial differences resulting from the choice of patient population for analysis should be the subject of explicit discussion.*

As mentioned before, it is therefore advantageous to ensure that compliance is similar across the treatment groups, since differential compliance can lead to seemingly contradictory results. It also means that any differences in treatment effects or safety parameters that might be caused by differences in compliance need to be carefully explored. To do this, you need enough granularity in the compliance data to analyse the effect. In practice, this means tablet counts, but also quality of self-administration where appropriate, electronic records of treatment administration if possible, electronic diaries or other means of recording that medication has been taken.

Of the two analyses, the ITT concept is the most widely accepted among statisticians and regulators (although some medical researchers question this). There are several reasons why ITT is used. First, it is a pragmatic comparison of treatment policies in clinical practice, in which non-compliance is common. Second, ITT is the only analysis that compares randomized treatment groups. When patients are removed from the trial, those that remain are often a non-comparable subset. For example, patients who receive active treatment may withdraw due to side-effects, whereas patients given a placebo may withdraw due to lack of any effect. In many cases, patients do not fare badly as a result of non-compliance, but rather do not comply as a result of faring badly. Peduzzi *et al.* (1993) present a real example of bias resulting from the exclusion of non-compliant patients.

It is true that ITT analysis underestimates the true treatment effect that would arise if the treatment were taken as prescribed. However, it is also true that few treatments will ever be taken exactly as prescribed! Consequently, the actual treatment effect observed in practice will, by definition, be different (usually less) than the theoretical effect that would be obtained in principle. The underestimation of the (theoretical) treatment effect as produced by ITT is in a sense a bias, yet is a predictable bias, and the conclusion of a treatment difference from an ITT analysis will be more convincing to sceptics. On the other hand, where patient populations are suspected of non-comparability, it is unclear how to interpret any findings.

There is one situation in which the ITT principle is challenged in analyses of efficacy, and this is in the increasingly encountered equivalence and non-inferiority trials. In these trials, the object is to show a new treatment to be 'the same as' (equivalence) or 'as good as' (non-inferiority) some control therapy. Since the ITT approach typically gives diluted estimates of treatment effect, non-compliance can lead to erroneous conclusions that treatments are more similar than they truly are. Regulatory guidelines require that per protocol analyses should be used alongside (and on an equal footing with) the ITT analysis in such trials, again requiring consistency in their findings.

The CONSORT statement makes no mention of compliance for safety analyses, and industry-sponsored trials rarely consider non-compliance in depth when assessing safety outcomes, in accordance with the ICH E9 (1998) guidelines:

> *For the overall safety and tolerability assessment, the set of subjects to be summarised is usually defined as those subjects who received at least one dose of the investigational drug.*

In other words, anything other than total non-compliance is often ignored when assessing safety. This issue is seldom discussed, yet it is important: Urquhart and de Klerk (1998) provide a sobering overview of the impact of non-compliance on safety (and efficacy), and argue persuasively that the manner in which compliance is commonly assessed and accounted for is inadequate. The reader is referred to this source for a fuller discussion.

From all of this, one thing is certain – those designing and interpreting clinical trials must have a clear understanding of which objectives the trial addresses and what the treatment comparisons mean. Both sets of analyses provide useful information when correctly interpreted.

Sample size considerations in the presence of non-compliance

Non-compliance impacts on the sample size requirements for both ITT and per protocol analyses. In ITT analyses, non-compliance leads to a decreased treatment effect and might also make patient response less homogeneous, thereby increasing the anticipated standard deviation. It is therefore prudent to calculate the required sample size using an overestimate of the standard deviation, and moreover it is essential to assume a more modest treatment effect than would be seen under perfect compliance. The estimated treatment effect is undiminished for per protocol comparisons, but since non-compliant patients are excluded here, the sample size requirement is again increased. This adjustment is simple enough: if n patients are required to ensure that the study has adequate power, and a proportion p are non-compliant, then the re-estimated sample size is n/p. For instance, if data from 100 patients are required but only 80 per cent of patients comply with treatment, then 100/0.8 = 125 patients are needed to achieve this, since 80 per cent of 125 is 100.

Many clinical trials explicitly calculate sample size on the basis of the per protocol analysis. This is acceptable practice, so long as the estimated treatment effect in the ITT comparison has also taken into account any impact of non-compliance.

Statistical modelling of non-compliance

There are sound reasons why the intention-to-treat analysis continues to be the approach of choice within clinical trials. Nonetheless, it is still of interest to have knowledge of the underlying (hypothetical) treatment effect, particularly if the trial produces unexpected findings that require thorough explanation. Compliance-adjusted analyses can also offer an estimate of the 'best achievable effect'. For example, a patient who is fully intent on complying with any medication may wish to know the benefit of the act of taking the treatment, as opposed to knowing what happens among patients as a whole.

Several statistical models have been proposed to account for compliance. However, it is important to recognize their drawbacks. First, they require a good quality of compliance data, which is time-consuming and adds expense. Although from a purely financial point of view, the cost of extra patients to differentiate a smaller treatment difference may be lower than some forms of expensive compliance monitoring techniques, it is also worth noting than improving compliance may also improve the treatment effect, therefore reducing the number of patients needed. Such an approach also brings the trial treatment closer to a disease management approach that may be used post-registration. Ideally, the trial should implement exactly that regime. Second, the complexity of statistical models hinders their interpretation by the non-mathematically minded reader, to whom these are 'black box methods'. Third, all methods make assumptions regarding compliance and its relationship to withdrawal or treatment allocation, which may be untrue or even untestable. Finally, at the time of writing, the applicability of such methods is limited by a lack of availability of statistical software. These approaches are therefore far from straightforward and should be used and interpreted with care.

The potential and the problems of methods for dealing with non-compliance are illustrated by the three proposed approaches below. We focus on the estimation of efficacy rather than safety, as does almost all of the methodology to date.

Pocock and Abdalla (1998) illustrated a simple method of exploring the relationship between effect size and compliance in a placebo-controlled trial in obesity. In this analysis, compliance was measured from plasma concentration of the active drug and its metabolite: the association between this marker and percentage weight loss was displayed graphically and a regression analysis performed, revealing a clear negative relationship between the two (that is, a greater weight reduction in more compliant patients). This method is simple and easy to apply, and any marker for treatment compliance can be used in this way. However, this association will invariably be confounded with other factors, and cannot be assumed causal.

Rubin (1998) proposed a method of analysing superiority trials in which an experimental treatment is compared to a control, and where non-compliance with experimental therapy is known. From this, a permutation-based method can be derived to test whether the treatment would be effective in those patients who would be compliant. Since it is unknown which patients in the control group would comply with the experimental therapy, this is estimated by multiple imputation methods from the patients' responses. It is assumed that patients who are non-compliant with experimental therapy would fare equally with control therapy.

White and Goetghebeur (1998) approached compliance in a different manner, using the approach of Robins and Tsiatis (1991) to test the sensitivity of a trial's results to non-compliance. A clinical trial of hypertension in elderly patients was re-analysed, incorporating the non-compliance observed in around half of the patients. Several aspects of non-compliance were investigated, including the taking of both, or neither, study treatments. The re-analysis assessed how large an effect was needed to overturn the treatment effect observed from the original ITT analysis. On this basis, they were able to conclude that no plausible effect of non-compliance could explain the apparent treatment benefit. This approach, in particular, is powerful in validating the scientific integrity of conclusions drawn from a trial.

Summary

The development of new methodology to adjust for the effects of non-compliance is an ongoing process, and has already yielded useful (if sometimes controversial) approaches to addressing compliance. It can be informative to investigate the relationship between compliance and outcome, since this can help understand any unusual trial results, assess robustness of the findings, identify potential problems with the process of undergoing treatment, and offer an estimate of the true underlying treatment effect. At the same time, as we have seen elsewhere in this chapter, compliance-adjusted treatment effects do not reflect the real-life situation when you are trying to determine whether a treatment is effective enough in a population to be registered. In this case, the best estimate of a treatment's effect is based not on what the treatment might offer, but rather on what a treatment decision has been shown to achieve in practice. Alternatively, when trying to make investment decisions, proof-of-concept decisions, or attempting to measure the individual benefit that any single patient might expect from a medication, the true underlying treatment effect is the most appropriate.

COMPLIANCE AS A PRIMARY ENDPOINT

Clinical trials that focus on compliance as a primary endpoint do so for a variety of reasons, the most common of which are as follows:

- To determine the best posology of the product – that is, to assess the optimal dose and frequency and/or to determine the best formulation for the product – to get the highest and most effective exposure of the patient to the medicine.
- To improve the effectiveness of the treatment regime to reduce the recurrence of a condition necessitating expensive acute care.
- To encourage patients to persevere with a treatment to get the best effect, either to finish a course of therapy, to cover a high-risk period effectively, to continue preventive medication even when the patients are feeling well, or for some other reason.
- To improve repeat sales and reduce wastage of the medicine.
- To demonstrate the best mix of approaches within a disease management programme.

In general these trials are carried out after a therapy has been registered and may be sponsored by the pharmaceutical company or by individuals within the healthcare system. Although these two different sets of sponsors look at compliance to therapy through different lenses, and thus have a differing focus, the actual tools, information and outcomes they measure are essentially the same, as are the final desired outcomes. For many years, formulation changes have formed the backbone of this sort of research. Compliance is improved if a patient has only to take one pill per day rather than three types of medicine four times a day. Once a day is harder to comply with than, say, a skin patch self-administered every week, or ultimately depot injections given by a healthcare professional (Linn, 2003). In recent times, although these more traditional approaches are still commonly studied, modern trials have had a broader spectrum of objectives, from measuring the effectiveness of an individual tool for increasing or measuring compliance right through to multifactor disease management programmes. The trials also target activities that occur in both the traditional healthcare setting of the hospital or clinic and the 'at home' setting. This is in recognition of the fact that the patients' treatment regimes are delivered 99 per cent of the time by themselves or immediate – usually family – carers, in their own home, which in turn means that the greatest opportunity for effecting the regime is in the 'at home' setting.

Trials generally fall into five categories, which are outlined below.

Trials of sensors in drug delivery equipment

The basic premise here is to count and date electronically the number of doses administered. The commonest tool is a microchip in a drug delivery device – typically an inhaler, nasal spray, syringe or suchlike. Also popular are chips in medicine bottle tops to monitor when they are opened, and blister pack or foil wrap 'holders' that count when they are opened to gain access to the medicine. These systems at their most basic provide nothing more than the data on when the drug was accessed. They usually tell you nothing about whether the patient actually took the medicine, threw it down the toilet or out of the window. They *will* reduce the incidence of patients dumping medicines in the car park, as the chip will show the doses all being accessed at the same time just before a trial visit. Clearly, these tools are most effective if the data are used in real time by the treating health professionals to remind the patient to take their medication as prescribed and to let the patient know that their poor compliance is visible (Bogen and Apter, 2004; Kohler, 2004; Iqbal *et al.*, 2004).

Physician aids to improve prescribing

These could be termed epidemiological compliance – ensuring that the greatest amount of treatment is taken by a population as a whole, not by an individual patient. Clearly, the first step in ensuring the right amount of medication is delivered to a patient is to ensure that it is correctly prescribed in the first place. Studies in this area cover bedside diagnostic and prescribing aids utilizing Personal Digital Assistants (PDA)s (Cannon, 2004; Koop and Mosges, 2002), treatment guidelines and algorithms being presented to physicians whilst using the clinic prescribing application on the desktop computer (Filippi *et al.*, 2003; Murray *et al.*, 2004; Yates *et al.*, 2001) and even physician training (Bryne *et al.*, 2004) to ensure the greatest implementation of best practices.

Patient reminders

These include the use of all mobile communication technology – SMS text, e-mails, wireless web pages and so on, which are dealt with in detail in Chapter 10 by Bill Byrom and David Stein. There are also trials utilizing Internet-based patient self-reporting of drug administration. These are based on the concept of giving the patient responsibility for the recording process, but in a more formal way than a diary, aiming to encourage accuracy. This is particularly helpful in studies on population kinetics in large phase III trials. There may not be enough data to collect to justify a PDA for the patient, and a device that records the dose access may not be practical, but reasonable accuracy of dose timings relative to blood sampling is critical for the result (Vrijens and Goetghebeur, 2004). Finally, there are also the devices that incorporate a reminder to access the medication, mentioned in the first section of this chapter (see also Buckwalter *et al.*, 2004). An example might be an alarm built into a medication dispenser that reminds the patient to take his or her medicine on time.

Patient feedback techniques

Thise are tools that requires some form of interaction or dialogue between the patient and the healthcare professionals or the tools and devices themselves. The simplest form is represented by a diabetic self-monitoring of the outcome of their therapy – a biofeedback process whereby the utilization of insulin can be titrated and refined in timing to gain the maximum diabetic control (Guerci *et al.*, 2003). More complex versions utilize a web-based system whereby the patients enter data into the system, which reacts with a series of possible responses either educational in nature – detailing the value of compliance and the effects of the illness – or logistical – for instance, organizing a meeting with a nurse, doctor or similar healthcare professional (Cherry *et al.*, 2002). More sophisticated feedback can be gained through a call-centre approach. A call centre manned by trained staff (for example, nurses) not only allows you to remind the patients in a timely way to take their medication, but can be very interactive in providing motivation, education, answering queries and so on (Grancelli *et al.*, 2003). The impact of home visits by either nurses or community pharmacists represents the next stage of feedback, with the patient being given information and treatment in the presence of a healthcare professional if possible, and the ability to answer whatever question crops up in a direct, personal, meaningful way (Cherry *et al.*, 2002; Grancelli *et al.*, 2003; Demyttenarere *et al.*, 2001).

Combinations of tools within disease management programmes

Combined systems tend to take the approaches investigated piecemeal as detailed above, and integrate them into disease management programmes to assess the 'bottom-line' effect. Many trials look at a set of possible interventions to improve compliance. However, most of these studies have a broader set of objectives to assess, such as the cost of care, incidence of recurrent illness and/or side-effects, quality of life, health economics and so on. These programmes often involve community-based staff visiting the patient at home either routinely or in response to some other data, as well as devices that measure access to medication, feedback techniques from devices or websites, call centres and so on (Cherry *et al.*, 2002).

Reviewing these trials, it is clear that in most cases any form of intervention is effective to a varying degree. This comes as no surprise, as any process that increases the attention paid to these types of outcome will inevitably lead to improvement. It is not always clear that the more complex approaches achieve better results, and therefore it is important when studying these data to look at the cost–benefit ratio achieved for the programme. What is clear is that the healthcare providers in Western countries have recognized that the centralized system of healthcare that they all tend to operate is overstretched and expensive, and may not give the best results. Adding in some element of ongoing interaction in the form of a simple device at one end of the scale, through to home nurse visits at the other end will not only tend to benefit the patients by increasing their exposure to the medicine and providing a set of readily defined community support systems, but also benefits both the pharmaceutical companies, by increasing the amount of prescribing and reducing wastage, and the healthcare delivery system in any particular country, by reducing cost of care and reducing demand on overutilized resources.

SUMMARY

We started with the premise that compliance is an important variable in clinical trials and that all stakeholders share similar goals in improving compliance. We discussed the intrinsic 'efficacy versus effectiveness' conflict – namely, the conflict between demonstrating the efficacy of a product through maximizing compliance and determining the realistic effect of the treatment in the normal clinical environment. The resolution of this dilemma is achieved by addressing the two separate questions across a development programme where both can be assessed in different clinical trials. This argument also demonstrates the value of cross-over learning between the two scenarios, where the tools used to enhance compliance in trials are applied in the real world in a disease management context, and vice versa.

We then looked at the tools and techniques utilized within trials to enhance compliance, by first assessing the causes of non-compliance, then the regulatory implications of non-compliance, and thus the best methods to combat it. We focused particularly on motivating the sites and the patients, and the effectiveness of the centralized healthcare system versus treating patients at home.

The statistical methods for dealing with compliance were outlined, mirroring the efficacy versus effectiveness conflict, and some different approaches to modelling compliance were discussed, providing a more sophisticated treatment of the issue in trial analysis.

The final section focused on trials designed to measure compliance as an endpoint in itself. Here the trials tend to reflect real life – usually focused on determining what the real-life compliance actually is and assessing different techniques to change compliance behaviour in the day-to-day medical care environment. In particular, we see the use of modern technology – especially mobile communications – to provide information to both patients and healthcare professionals, which can be used for feedback on the value of compliance; and the use of the disease management approach to provide a continual interaction with the patients in their home environment in order to keep the treatment at the front of their minds more regularly.

Compliance is key to the efficient use of healthcare resources. The better patients are treated the less they utilize the healthcare systems and the less they cost. This holds true even if more interactions between the patient and the system take place – either electronically or in person – implying that the healthcare system needs to undergo a fundamental paradigm shift towards complex, sophisticated disease management methodologies if it is to more effectively improve the overall health of the population.

REFERENCES

Blackwell, B. (1976), 'Treatment Adherence', *British Journal of Psychiatry*, **129**, pp. 513–31.

Blackwell, B. (1996), 'From Compliance to Alliance: A Quarter Century of Research', *Netherlands Journal of Medicine*, **48**, pp. 140–49.

Bogen, D. and Apter, A.J. (2004), 'Adherence Logger for a Dry Powder Inhaler: A New Device for Medical Adherence Research', *Journal of Clinical Immunology*, **11**(4), pp. 863–68.

Buckwalter, K.C., Wakefield, B.J., Hanna, B. and Lehmann, J. (2004), 'New Technology for Medication Adherence: Electronically Managed Dispensing System', *Journal of Gerontological Nursing*, **30**(7), pp. 5–8.

Bryne, M.K., Deane, F.P., Lambert, G. and Coombs, T. (2004), 'Enhancing Medication Adherence: Clinician Outcomes from the Medication Alliance Training Program', *Australia and New Zealand Journal of Psychiatry*, **38**(4), pp. 246–53.

Cannon, C.P. (2004), 'Utilisation of Guidelines and Computer Based Technology to Achieve Optimal Care in Atherothrombotic Vascular Disease', *Journal of Thrombosis and Thrombolysis*, **17**(1), pp. 45–49.

Cherry, J.C., Moffatt, T.P., Rodriguez, C. and Dryden, K. (2002), 'Diabetes Disease Management Program for an Indigenous Population Empowered by Telemedicine Technology', *Diabetes Technology and Therapeutics*, **4**(6), pp. 783–91.

Demyttenaere, K., Enzlin, P., Dewe, W., Boulanger, B., De Bie, J., De Troyer, W. and Mesters, P. (2001), 'Compliance with Antidepressants in a Primary Care Setting, 1: Beyond Lack of Efficacy and Adverse Events', *Journal of Clinical Psychiatry*, **62**, Suppl. 22, pp. 30–33.

Detailed Guidance on the Collection, Verification and Presentation of Adverse Reaction Reports Arising from Clinical Trials on Medicinal Products for Human Use, (2004), European Commission, Brussels, ENTR/F2/BL D(2003), April, at: http://eudract.emea.eu.int/docs/Detailed%20guidance%20collection%20of%20adverse%20events.pdf (accessed 2006).

Farup, P.G. (1992), 'Compliance with Anti-ulcer Medication During Short-term Healing Phase Clinical Trials', *Alimentary Pharmacology and Therapeutics*, (2), pp. 179–86.

Fayers, P.M., Hopwood, P., Harvey, A., Girling, D.J., Machin, D. and Stephens, R. (1997), 'Quality of Life Assessment in Clinical Trials – Guidelines and a Checklist for Protocol Writers: The U.K. Medical Research Council Experience', *European Journal of Cancer*, **33**(1), pp. 20–28.

Filippi, A., Sabatini, A., Badioli, L., Samani, F., Mazzaglia, G. and Catapano, A. (2003), 'Effects of an Automated Electronic Reminder in Changing the Anti Platelet Drug Prescribing Behaviour among Italian General Practitioners in Diabetic Patients: An Intervention Trial', *Diabetes Care*, **26**(5), pp. 1497–500.

Gitlin, M.J., Cochran, S.D. and Jamison, K.R. (1989), 'Maintenance Lithium Treatment: Side Effects and Compliance', *Journal of Clinical Psychiatry*, **50**, pp. 127–31.

Grancelli, H., Varini, S., Ferrante, D., Schwartzman, R., Zambrano, C., Soifer, S., Nul, D. and Doval, H., GESICA Investigators (2003), 'Randomised Trial of Telephone Intervention in Chronic Heart Failure (DIAL): Study Design and Preliminary Observations', *Journal of Cardiac Failure*, **9**(3), pp. 172–79.

Greenberg, R.N. (1984), 'Overview of Patient Compliance with Medication Dosing: A Literature Review', *Clinical Therapy*, **6**(5), pp. 592–99.

Guerci, B., Drouin, P., Grange, V., Bougneres, P., Fontaine, P., Kerlan, V., Passa, P., Thivolet, Ch., Vialettes, B. and Charbonnel, B., ASIA Group, (2003), 'Self-monitoring of Blood Glucose Significantly Improves Metabolic Control in Patients with Type II Diabetes Mellitus: The Auto Surveillance Intervention Active (ASIA) Study', *Diabetes and Metabolism*, **29**(6), pp. 587–94.

ICH (International Conference on the Harmonisation of Technical Requirements for Registration of Pharmaceuticals for Human Use) (1995), 'Structure and Content of Clinical Study Reports', ICH topic E3, Step 4 at: http://www.ich.org/1995.

ICH (International Conference on the Harmonisation of Technical Requirements for Registration of Pharmaceuticals for Human Use) (1998), 'Statistical Principles for Clinical Trials', ICH topic E9, Step 4 at: http://www.ich.org/1998.

Iqbal, S., Ritson, I., Denyer, J. and Everard, M.L. (2004), 'Drug Delivery and Adherence in Young Children', *Pediatric Pulmonology*, **37**(4), pp. 311–17.

Kirscht, J.P. and Rosenstock, I.M. (1980), 'Patients' Problems in Following the Recommendations of Health Experts', in G.C. Stone, F. Cohen and M.E. Adler (eds), *Health Psychology: A Handbook*, San Francisco: Jossey-Bass, pp. 189–215.

Kohler, D. (2004), 'The Novoliser: Overcoming Inherent Problems of Dry Powder Inhalers', *Respiratory Medicine*, **98**, Suppl. A, pp. S17–21.

Koop, A. and Mosges, R. (2002), 'The Use of Handheld Computers in Clinical Trials', *Controlled Clinical Trials*, **23**(5), pp. 469–80.

Leppik, I.E. (1990), 'How to Get Patients with Epilepsy to Take their Medication: The Problem of Non-compliance', *Postgraduate Medicine*, **88**, pp. 253–56.

Linn, E.S. (2003), 'Progress in Contraception: New Technology', *International Journal of Fertility and Women's Medicine*, **48**(4), pp. 182–91.

Moher, D., Schulz, K.F. and Altman, D.G. for the CONSORT Group (2001), 'The CONSORT Statement: Revised Recommendations for Improving the Quality of Reports of Parallel-group Randomised Trials' at: http://www.consort-statement.org/2001.

Murray, M.D., Harris, L.E., Overhage, J.M., Zhou, X.H., Eckert, G.J., Smith, F.E., Buchanan, N.N., Wolinsky, F.D., McDonald, C.J. and Tierney, W.M. (2004), 'Failure of Computerised Treatment Suggestions to Improve Health Outcomes in Patients with Uncomplicated Hypertension: Results of a Randomised Controlled Trial', *Pharmacotherapy*, **24**(3), pp. 324–37.

Myers, E.D. and Branthwaite, A. (1992), 'Outpatient Compliance with Antidepressant Medication', *British Journal of Psychiatry*, **160**, pp. 83–86.

Peduzzi, P., Wittes, J. and Detre, K. (1993), 'Analysis As-randomized and the Problem of Non-adherence: An Example from the Veterans' Affairs Randomized Trial of Coronary Artery Bypass Surgery', *Statistics in Medicine*, **12**, pp. 1185–95.

Pocock, S. and Abdalla, M. (1998). 'The Hope and Hazards of Using Compliance Data in Randomized Controlled Trials', *Statistics in Medicine*, **17**, pp. 303–17.

Pullar, T., Birtwell, A.J., Wiles, P.G. *et al.* (1988), 'Use of a Pharmacologic Indicator to Compare Compliance with Tablets Taken Once, Twice or Three Times Daily', *International Journal of Clinical Pharmacology and Therapeutics*, **44**, pp. 540–45.

Robins, J.M. and Tsiatis, A.A. (1991), 'Correcting for Non-compliance in Randomized Trials Using Rank Preserving Structural Failure Time Models', *Communications in Statistics – Theory and Methods*, **20**, pp. 2609–31.

Rubin, D.B. (1998), 'More Powerful Randomization-based P-values in Double-blind Trials with Non-compliance', *Statistics in Medicine*, **17**, pp. 371–85.

Shaw, E. (1986), 'Lithium Non-compliance', *Psychiatric Annals*, **16**(S10), pp. 583–88.

Simmons, M.S., Nides, M.A. and Rand, C.S. (2000), 'Unpredictability of Deception in Compliance with Physician-prescribed Bronchodilator Inhaler Use in a Clinical Trial', *Chest*, **118**, pp. 290–95.

Spector, S.L., Kinsman, R., Mawhinney, H., Siegel, S.C., Rachelefsky, G.S., Katz, R.M. and Rohr, A.S. (1986), 'Compliance of Patients with Asthma with an Experimental Aerosolized Medication: Implications for Controlled Clinical Trials', *Journal of Allergy and Clinical Immunology*, **77**(1), Pt 1, pp. 65–70.

Stone, A.A., Shiffman, S., Schwartz, J.E., Broderick, J.E. and Hufford, M.R. (2002), 'Patient Non-compliance with Paper Diaries', *British Medical Journal*, **324**(7347), pp. 1193–94.

Taggart, A.J., Johnson, G.D. and McDevitt, D.G. (1981), 'Does the Frequency of Daily Dosage Influence Compliance with Digoxin Therapy?', *British Journal of Clinical Pharmacology*, **1**, pp. 31–34.

Urquhart, J. and de Klerk, E. (1998), 'Contending Paradigms for the Interpretation of Data on Patient Compliance with Therapeutic Drug Regimens', *Statistics in Medicine*, **17**, pp. 251–67.

Vrijens, B. and Goetghebeur, E. (2004), 'Electronic Monitoring in Drug Intakes Can Reduce Bias and Improve Precision in Pharmacokinetic/Pharmacodynamic Population Studies', *Statistics in Medicine*, **23**(4), pp. 531–44.

White, I.R. and Goetghebeur, E.J.T. (1998), 'Clinical Trials Comparing Two Treatment Policies: Which Aspects of the Treatment Policies Make a Difference?', *Statistics in Medicine*, **17**, pp. 319–39.

Yates, S., Annis, L., Pippins, J. and Walden, S. (2001), 'Does a Lipid Clinic Increase Compliance with National Cholesterol Education Program Treatment Guidelines? Report of a Case Matched Controlled Study', *Southern Medical Journal*, **94**(9), pp. 907–909.

CHAPTER 9

The Role of Pharma's Field-based Professionals in Patient Compliance

Dr Jane Y. Chin, PhD

PATIENT COMPLIANCE CROSSES BORDERS AND DISEASE STATES

Patient compliance rates may differ between nations – patients in developing countries often being less compliant than those in developed countries – but compliance is crossing socioeconomic borders to challenge both developed and developing countries (WHO, 2001). Two years after the World Health Organization (WHO) published its *Policy for Action*, the international organization published *Adherence to Long-term Therapies: Evidence for Action* (WHO, 2003) and recommended a multidisciplinary approach in improving patient compliance. C. Everett Koop, the former US Surgeon General said, 'Drugs don't work if people don't take them', and in 2003 the *Wall Street Journal* labelled patient compliance as the 'Real Drug Problem' in the United States, claiming that 'rich, highly educated people are just as likely not to take their medicine as poor or less-educated people' (cited in Marcus, 2003).

Patient compliance, also known as patient adherence, was defined as 'the extent to which a person's behaviour – taking medication, following a diet, and/or executing lifestyle changes – corresponds with agreed recommendations from a health care provider' by the WHO's Adherence Project (WHO, 2003). Patient compliance rates can also differ between disease states: patients with diseases that require chronic administration of medication are often less compliant than those requiring short-term drug therapy. For example, poor patient compliance is an obstacle in the successful management of diabetes and depression after the initial medical intervention. Even acute conditions are not immune to poor patient compliance. Poor patient compliance contributes to the increasing antibiotic resistance in respiratory tract infections: patients may not take the complete course of antibiotics because they are feeling better or they may forget to take an antibiotic if the regimen requires multiple doses per day.

Patient compliance is increasingly recognized as a problem extending beyond following physicians' instructions. The World Health Organization has identified five dimensions of patient compliance that require active participation from each dimension's stakeholders. These dimensions are:

- health system and healthcare team factors
- social/economic factors
- therapy-related factors
- patient-related factors
- condition-related factors (WHO, 2003).

The role of physicians in patient compliance continues to be emphasized: physicians are encouraged to proactively address patient compliance from both a process standpoint and a relationship standpoint. Physicians can systematically assess and address compliance issues at the point of disbursing the therapeutic regimen to the patient, by managing patient expectations up-front and explaining potential side-effects. They then assume a collaborative stance by giving the patients information on how they can manage expected side-effects and by involving caregivers and the patient's family members (Jaret, 2001).

Electronic patient diaries have become a staple in the armoury for enhancing patient compliance. Other tools include devices that monitor pill disbursement and provide an objective measure of patient compliance, and electronic devices that are placed in pill caps and send information about a patient's actual compliance with the medication. Technology, however, will not replace the relationship between patient and physician. The recent terminological proclivity towards 'adherence' suggests recognition of the patient as an active member in his or her own disease management, as well as an emphasis on a commitment and relationship between the patient and the physician. A patient who perceives the physician as caring may be more likely to adhere. Today's litigious environment demands that physicians be vigilant about patient compliance by proactively communicating and building trust with their patients and patients' caregivers. Physicians cannot be complacent about patient compliance and are reminded to engage patients and patients' caregivers in a dialogue about adhering to a therapeutic regimen. Inconsistencies in patient compliance can often surface when patients are probed further (Elliot, 2004).

Patient compliance continues to be a concern because modern-day physicians have less time to spend communicating and building a relationship with each patient. Moreover, compliance implementation has generally focused on patient-related factors and a unidimensional approach. Even though it is agreed that patient compliance is important and even in the context of technological aids, results have not met expectations.

THE PHARMACEUTICAL INDUSTRY AND PATIENT COMPLIANCE

The World Health Organization has called for a multidisciplinary approach in improving patient compliance that involves health professionals, researchers, health planners and policy-makers. Patient compliance with a medication regimen directly affects the effectiveness and safety of that medication – factors in the formation of physicians' perceptions about a medication or treatment regimen. In turn, physicians' perceptions about a treatment influence their prescribing behaviour. As manufacturers of therapeutics, pharmaceutical companies have an interest in patient compliance and can be a critical contributor in a multidisciplinary approach to the issue.

Pharmaceutical companies can offer significant research- and education-related resources for improving patient compliance. A recent conference workshop on patient compliance targeted at pharmaceutical industry constituents identified common implementation barriers to patient compliance and common elements to good compliance programmes. Industry best practices included partnering with healthcare providers and motivating them to focus on patient compliance, thinking from the patient or end-user perspective, and involving nurses in managing patient compliance (Roner, 2004).

Partnering with physicians is important because physicians often overestimate their patients' compliance to medication regimens. As nurses and physician assistants (PAs) are increasingly becoming patients' primary points of contact for information following physician diagnoses, industry–practitioner partnership should also extend to nurses and PAs. The pharmaceutical industry's field-based teams are poised to facilitate industry–practitioner partnerships that enhance patient compliance. Medical science liaison teams (MSLs, also referred as 'medical liaisons') are field-based pharmaceutical professionals whose role is clinically driven and distinct and separate from that of field-based pharmaceutical sales representatives.

AN OVERVIEW OF PHARMA'S MEDICAL SCIENCE LIAISON TEAMS

Medical liaisons are therapeutic specialists and, in the United States, are generally organized under the Medical Affairs or comparable scientific department. Medical liaisons often have advanced scientific training and hold doctorate degrees in life sciences, a trend that has gained prominence in today's intensely scrutinized pharmaceutical environment (Chin, 2003, 2005a). Medical liaison programmes have established an integral foothold in the pharmaceutical company's product life-cycle management, based on MSLs' role in the positive positioning of a company's therapeutic focus.

Medical liaisons participate in a product's pre- and post-launch activities, cultivating relationships with recognized thought-leaders in a therapeutic area. The industry's relationship with medical thought-leaders, also known as key opinion leaders or KOLs, is a symbiotic collaboration towards understanding disease states and appropriate drug utilisation, and contributing to the scientific body of evidence for a therapeutic product.

In recent years, MSLs have become primary points of contact between scientific pioneers and pharmaceutical companies (Chin, 2001).

MEDICAL SCIENCE LIAISONS IN CLINICAL RESEARCH

Medical liaisons facilitate clinical research projects between investigators and pharmaceutical companies, and have an active role in the pharmaceutical organization's clinical development approaches in a given therapeutic area. Synergy between all stakeholders in a clinical trial can have an impact on attaining study milestones and make a difference to a company's first-to-market advantage for a therapeutic. Therefore, MSL teams help maintain productive collaboration between pharmaceutical development scientists, clinical research personnel, clinical investigators and research coordinators.

Medical liaisons engage clinical investigators in a dialogue about the scientific approach for a research concept and participate in discussions spanning study design and side-effect management. In an investigator-sponsored study (also known as investigator-initiated trial or IIT), the clinical investigator contacts the MSL with a research concept. In a company-sponsored study, the MSL approaches potential investigators with the research opportunity. In the case of an IIT, the investigator submits a letter of intent (LOI) to the pharmaceutical organization via the MSL. If the MSL determines that the concept should generate a high level of interest from the company, the liaison compiles an investigator's package that includes the LOI, the investigator's curriculum vitae (CV), supporting information about the investigator's ability to successfully conduct the study and appropriate disclosure forms. This package is submitted to the company and queued for review by the company's medical review committee. During the medical review, the MSL serves as the investigator's champion.

If the medical review committee approves the investigator's concept, the investigator will be invited to submit a complete clinical trial protocol. The MSL remains the investigator's main point of contact throughout this process, and actively participates in supporting the investigator's effort by providing necessary drug information. The MSL will also review the clinical protocol for completeness of the study calendar (clinical study plan), side-effect management approaches and informed consent. The MSL may also speak with research staff at the potential study site to assess the clinical research experience of the investigator's staff and available mechanisms for enrolling patients. Medical liaisons help ensure timely completion of clinical studies and encourage investigators to submit clinical study data for publication and presentation at scientific venues (Chin, 2004, 2005b).

MEDICAL SCIENCE LIAISONS IN CLINICAL EDUCATION

Medical liaisons are often viewed as field-based extensions of a pharmaceutical organization's clinical research and medical information functions. One of MSLs' responsibilities is to foster collaborative relationships between the pharmaceutical company and medical thought-leaders, to serve as the 'face' of the organization, thereby enhancing the company's visibility in a therapeutic area. Dissemination of scientific information is the main approach through which MSLs cultivate relationships with medical thought-leaders, and this is the clinical education function of the MSL role.

Medical liaisons communicate information from medical thought-leaders to the pharmaceutical company and complete the circuit of active scientific information exchange between the industry and the medical community. Scientific information exchange may occur through various avenues, from informal, one-to-one interactions between a MSL and a medical thought-leader to formal clinical presentations to a healthcare audience. Medical liaisons present clinical study updates, facilitate round-table discussions of relevant therapeutic topics with physicians, and participate in thought-leader advisory boards. They also conduct speaker training, in which the liaison works with a physician who has expressed interest in discussing a company's therapeutic agent on that pharmaceutical company's behalf.

In addition, medical liaisons support other pharmaceutical field-based teams, including pharmaceutical sales representatives and managed care account managers. In this regard, they sometimes serve as a support to other field-based functions, reactively providing and clarifying scientific information, including responses to unsolicited requests for off-label information from healthcare practitioners. Managed care account managers often recruit their medical liaison colleagues to present clinical product data to support formulary and contracting initiatives within an institution or a network of institutions. At a national level, medical liaison teams provide clinical information to medical thought-leaders who establish treatment guidelines and policies for a disease.

Given the role of medical liaison teams in facilitating clinical research and disseminating scientific information between pharmaceutical companies and physicians, medical liaisons can become an integral component of the pharmaceutical industry's effort to address patient compliance. During a product's clinical development phase, medical liaisons interact with clinical investigators and can serve as an information conduit between the pharmaceutical organization and researchers. As the product becomes commercialized, medical liaisons can provide education and clinical support to physicians and support staff. They are therefore poised to keep patient compliance at the forefront of therapeutic intervention.

FACTORING PATIENT COMPLIANCE INTO CLINICAL DEVELOPMENT

Clinical trials are highly controlled milieus for dissecting the safety and efficacy profiles of a therapeutic agent. Human subjects enrolled in a clinical trial are carefully monitored by investigators and research personnel, and follow-up appointments are built into the clinical study plan. However, patient compliance is a recognized problem even within this highly controlled, clinical trial environment (see also Chapter 8 by Graham Wylie and his colleagues), Nevertheless, patient compliance is a key factor in successfully developing and marketing a drug. The cost of drug development is approaching US$1 billion per marketed drug, and clinical trials have become formidable investments, requiring the enrolment of large numbers of patients and often involving many countries.

Poor patient compliance can risk the very clinical trial outcome required for drug approval, by misattributing patient compliance-related outcomes to a drug's safety or efficacy profile. This in turn contributes to the cost of drug development, which factors in the cost of development failures for every drug development success.

Once a therapeutic agent is commercialized and available to the community, drug safety and efficacy become unpredictable, because patients in a 'real-world' situation may not be as compliant as patients in a clinical trial setting. When the therapeutic regimen is complex or when the therapeutic regimen becomes part of the patient's daily routine, patient compliance becomes a critical issue in the success of therapeutic intervention and in ensuring patient safety. Medical and healthcare advances are transforming once-fatal diseases into chronic conditions that are often controlled through polypharmacy. Patients must now manage their own conditions for prolonged periods, often for the rest of their lives. Inadequate management of chronic diseases can lead to complications and co-morbidities with a significant healthcare burden; diabetes is such an example. Therefore, the role of patient compliance will only increase in the context of adequate disease management and controlling burgeoning healthcare costs.

Factoring patient compliance into the clinical trial plan helps ensure that a therapeutic is successfully marketed in a community setting, just as judicious study design and efficient research processes help ensure the timely completion of a clinical trial. Medical liaisons are deployed as local research contacts for clinical investigators to address research concept- and education-related issues surrounding a clinical trial. Clinical development presents medical liaisons with an opportunity to address patient compliance factors with principal investigators, so that the therapeutic regimen and study plan are designed with patient compliance in mind. Medical liaisons can pay particular attention to the informed consent document, and make sure that the information given is comprehensive *and* comprehensible. The investigator should also discuss with the patient what support and resources are available during the clinical trial should the patient have any questions or concerns.

Therapy-related factors that affect adherence include the complexity of the medical regimen, the duration of treatment, previous treatment failures, frequent changes in treatment, the immediacy of beneficial effects, side-effects and available medical support to manage side-effects (WHO, 2003). If the desired patient compliance downstream of clinical development is to be achieved, these factors should be considered as early as the drug formulation stage. Drug formulation dictates how a drug would be administered, how often the drug would be administered and potential side-effects due to the route of administration and drug formulation.

Medical liaisons learn about patient experiences with a therapeutic approach by interacting with medical thought-leaders and can channel this perspective to the pharmaceutical company. If compliance issues are likely to arise with a particular intervention, these issues can be identified early in development, and the company can customize product development to minimize or eliminate a known patient compliance issue. Treatment that requires significant alteration of habit of a patient's daily life or has an impact on a quality of life (QoL) that the patient considers important will risk a low patient compliance rate, because the patient may not be able to immediately modify habits or adjust to the expectations demanded by a therapeutic regimen.

Because medical liaisons are field-based, these clinical professionals are frequently the first to learn about emerging concerns in patient compliance that pharmaceutical marketers may not immediately be aware of. QoL-related compliance factors are such examples. In the field of psychiatry, certain classes of antidepressants are widely known to cause sexual dysfunction in depressed patients, which predisposes patients to poor compliance. Healthcare practitioners are now addressing QoL issues, such as sexual function in patients, in managing side-effects from antidepressant therapy, and pharmaceutical marketers are being made aware of patients' self-management of such QoL concerns (patients frequently stopped taking their medication or took 'drug holidays').

Diabetes management provides another example of the role medical liaisons can play in alerting pharmaceutical companies to patient compliance concerns. Pharmaceutical marketers of the thiazolidinedione class of oral anti-diabetics had addressed oedema as a side effect because of the potential for oedema to precipitate coronary and pulmonary events. However, medical liaisons in the diabetes field have heard from their physicians that some patients are concerned with a 'quality of life' factor behind non-compliance due to oedema. Some patients who are unhappy with the cosmetic effects of oedema stop taking their medication.

Medical liaisons in the oncology field may become aware of compliance issues with complicated interventions common with cancer therapeutics. For example, the continuous infusion of an oncology drug may be required to ensure steady dosing of a therapeutic. However, continuous infusion is inconvenient for patients if therapeutic intervention must occur over a span of several days. Additionally, complications such as infection or allergic reaction at the infusion site can occur with continuous intravenous administration. Product development scientists may weigh the rate of patient compliance in an intervention requiring continuous intravenous infusion with a formulation that requires a single infusion dosing, or with oral formulations that require patients to take a pill several times a day. A regimen with thrice-daily or twice-daily dosing may not garner the same level of patient compliance as a once-daily regimen, but may have more favourable patient compliance rates than a continuous intravenous infusion regimen or a single infusion dosing regimen (see also Chapter 7 by Akira Kusai).

Even formulation strategies may be oversimplifying the complexity of patient compliance. The use of oral agents in cancer therapy is an example. Although oral agents appear more convenient than intravenous administration of cancer therapy, the reimbursement debate seemed to have gained more attention than the impact that oral anti-cancer agents may have on patient compliance (Thomas *et al.*, 2000). Patient compliance in cancer therapy can affect the patient's chance of survival. Unlike infusion cancer therapies, patients will probably self-administer an oral anti-cancer agent and may not be adequately prepared to manage side-effects should they arise. Many cancer patients may prefer to receive infusion therapy at an oncology clinic and have access to healthcare support, rather than self-administer a cancer therapeutic at home. Patient expectations of how their diseases should be managed will also influence patient compliance. With advances in cancer therapeutics where oncologists are beginning to shift from an acute cancer treatment approach to a chronic cancer management approach, cancer patients will see an emphasis in self-management of cancer symptoms and even on self-administering cancer agents. Arguably, as cancer becomes a chronic condition, patient compliance attitudes and behaviour may begin to resemble those of chronic diseases like diabetes, asthma, and depression.

Medical liaisons are therefore exposed to patient preferences through dialogue with research investigators and physicians, and can communicate this information to their organization. Information that medical liaisons receive from the field on patient compliance trends, attitudes and behaviours for an interventionist approach help a pharmaceutical company make drug formulation decisions and design clinical trials that optimize its market positioning.

FACTORING PATIENT COMPLIANCE INTO CLINICAL EDUCATION

Medical liaison teams are becoming integrated into pharmaceutical companies' early brand-building efforts, contributing to early brand-building strategies and tactics in drug commercialization. Medical liaisons' role in clinical education is a component in pharmaceutical companies' brand-building efforts and their building of relationships with medical thought-leaders. As medical liaisons have a role in enhancing awareness of patient compliance during clinical development, they continue to have a role in maintaining patient compliance at the forefront of the minds of physicians, nurses and other healthcare professionals. Medical liaisons facilitate company-sponsored educational venues such as advisory boards and consultant meetings, and can incorporate discussions about patient compliance in these informational exchange platforms.

Since polypharmacy is the norm in managing complex and chronic conditions, medical liaisons partner with a healthcare team by providing product information and clinical education to physicians and members of the healthcare team. They do *not* necessarily confine discussions to the products they represent on their companies' behalf, because their value to physicians and healthcare teams comes from the way in which they serve as a disease state expert and a partner in disease management. For example, a marketed cancer therapeutic is known to affect lipid levels in patients taking the anti-cancer drug. To meet the clinical information needs of the oncology community, the company's medical liaisons will provide information on the cancer therapeutic as well as educating physicians and healthcare teams on lipid management and lipid dysfunction. In this case, patient compliance on a lipid management regimen is critical for the success of the oncology therapeutic.

Nurses are front-line health practitioners who can form close relationships with patients and also are first to hear of patients' fears and frustrations about a treatment, often being the first to learn about a patient's non-compliance due to quality-of-life concerns or factors not immediately visible to physicians. By interacting with patients and querying their perceptions of, and satisfaction with, the treatment, nurses are valuable drivers of patient compliance. They also directly educate patients on management of their conditions, answer patients' questions about a therapy or side-effects, and reassure patients who are fearful about their condition or the treatment. Medical liaisons can support nurses and healthcare staff by providing educational 'in-services' and inviting input from nurses and other members of the healthcare team. Medical liaisons can also provide nurses with additional resources and education that enhance the healthcare team's patient compliance effort, as well as channel feedback from nurses and the healthcare team about a therapeutic approach back to the pharmaceutical organization.

MEDICAL LIAISONS AND INDUSTRY'S PATIENT COMPLIANCE EFFORT

To begin integrating the medical liaison function into industry's effort to increase patient compliance, pharmaceutical companies need to build this expectation into the medical liaison job description and provide appropriate training for medical liaisons. Pharmaceutical companies rarely train medical liaisons in patient compliance, and, unless medical liaisons have had prior patient care experience, most will hand patient compliance issues back to physicians. Given the complexity of, and the multidimensional influences on, patient compliance, companies should incorporate patient compliance consideration and issues into disease state and product training for medical liaisons.

When medical liaisons conduct 'speaker training' and work with physicians who are interested in speaking about a product, pharmaceutical companies can incorporate patient compliance training into the speaker's presentation. Since the physician–patient relationship will remain the critical driver of patient compliance, pharmaceutical companies can help physicians assess patient compliance and advise on how to increase it. Given that a successful therapeutic intervention depends on patient compliance, issues affecting patient compliance with the company's drug should be discussed as part of speaker training. Similar consideration may be implemented in medical liaison-facilitated advisory boards and consultant meetings, where physicians can be encouraged to share their insights and suggestions for a therapeutic intervention. Advisory boards and consultant meetings also enable physicians to learn from their peers on best practices in increasing patient compliance for a therapeutic intervention.

Because patient compliance can translate into a commercial interest for the organization, medical liaisons may view patient compliance as a problem better addressed by marketing than by medical or scientific affairs. This perception must be addressed and changed before medical liaison teams can be successfully integrated in pharmaceutical companies' efforts to increase patient compliance. Patient compliance may be addressed as a clinical development issue, rather than a post-marketing issue, where compliance is critical in the integrity of clinical efficacy and safety data for a therapeutic. It is a significant factor in a product's market positioning, and companies that proactively identify patient compliance challenges during early clinical development are in a better position to steer the course of a product's development to ensure post-marketing success.

Pharmaceutical marketing and promotional practices are closely scrutinized in the United States, and medical liaisons' involvement in patient compliance should invite regulatory and ethical consideration. Since medical liaisons do not interact directly with patients, patient privacy concerns may not be immediate. Nevertheless, medical liaisons should be vigilant in helping physicians and healthcare teams maintain patient privacy when discussing patient compliance. Additionally, patient compliance assistance programmes have been identified by the Department of Health and Human Services' Office of Inspector General as posing a potential risk of kickback violations.[1] Such kickbacks are directed towards pharmaceutical companies' gathering feedback about patient compliance from physicians through advisory board and consultant meetings ('Compliance Program Guidance', 2003). Companies should regularly conduct internal audits to ensure that contracts with physicians are appropriately documented to satisfy the personal services safe harbour and that these venues are indeed legitimate in soliciting physicians' insight in patient compliance.

CONCLUSIONS

Patient compliance is a multidimensional, multinational and multidisease state problem. Pharmaceutical companies have the resources and commercial interest to proactively support the patient compliance effort by partnering with physicians and healthcare teams. Despite technological advances in enhancing patient compliance, physician–patient relationships remain the key driver of good patient compliance. Pharmaceutical companies can therefore aid physicians and healthcare staff by providing training and support towards enhanced patient compliance.

Since partnering with physicians remains an industry best practice for improving patient compliance, field-based medical professionals who regularly interface with physicians can play a role in industry–physician partnerships in improving patient compliance. Medical liaisons can facilitate clinical research and development and can provide information about patient compliance with a proposed therapeutic approach to the pharmaceutical company. This information enables the company to make product development decisions, such as formulation, even before drug commercialization. Once a drug is commercialized, medical liaisons can continue to raise awareness of patient compliance when interacting with physicians and healthcare providers.

The successful implementation of field-based medical liaison programmes into the industry's patient compliance efforts requires pharmaceutical companies to train medical liaisons on patient compliance, build the expectation of enhancing patient compliance into medical liaisons' clinical role, and set clear guidelines on medical liaison-facilitated educational venues to ensure regulatory compliance.

REFERENCES

Chin, J.Y. (2001), 'Medical Science Liaisons: An Overview', Medical Science Liaison Institute, available at: http://www.mslinstitute.com.

1. 'Kickback'= bribe. The term 'kickback' is used because, in the US codes of federal regulations (laws), the name of the law is the Anti-Kickback Statute.

Chin, J.Y. (2003), 'Medical Science Liaisons: Examining the Role, Revisited', *Medical Science Liaison Quarterly*, **1**(4), available at: http://www.msliq.com/mslstore/index.php?mainpage=index&cPath=23.

Chin, J.Y. (2004), 'Why Liaisons Lead to Clinical Trial Success', *Good Clinical Practice Journal*, **11**(1), available at: http://www.msliq.com/mslstore/index.php?mainpage=index&cPath=23.

Chin, J.Y. (2005a), 'MSLs: Off Label Promotion', *Pharmaceutical Executive*, January, available at: http://www.pharmexec.com/pharmexec/article/articleDetail.jsp?id=146598.

Chin, J.Y. (2005b), *Partnering with Key Opinion Leaders in Investigator-Initiated Trials*, ExL Pharma's Successful, Compliant Investigator-Initiated Trial Programs, Philadelphia, 10–11 February (Publication of Proceedings).

'Compliance Program Guidance for Pharmaceutical Manufacturers' (2003), *Federal Register*, **68**(86), 5 May/Notices, at: http://www.epa.gov/fedrgstr/EPAFR-CONTENTS/2003/May/Day-05/contents.htm.

Elliot, P.L. (2004), '4 Steps to Better Patient Compliance', *Medical Economics*, **81**(22), 19 November, pp. 30, 31–32.

Jaret, P. (2001), '10 Ways to Improve Patient Compliance', *Hippocrates*, **15**(2), available at: http://www.hippocrates.com.

Marcus, A.D. (2003), 'The Real Drug Problem: Forgetting to Take Them', *Wall Street Journal*, 21 October.

Roner, Lisa (2004), 'Barriers, Best Practices and Measuring ROI for Patient Compliance Programs', eyeforpharma's Patient Persistence, Compliance & Education Conference, Philadelphia, 19–20 October at: http://www.eyeforpharma.com/briefing/pcusawriteup.pdf.

Thomas, F.W. *et al.* (2000), 'Oral Chemotherapy, Cytostatic, and Supportive Care Agents: New Opportunities and Challenges', *Oncology Issues*, **15**(2), available at: http://www.accc-cancer.org/ONIS/onis_about.asp.

WHO (2001), 'Adherence to Long-term Therapies', World Health Organization at: http://www.who.int/chronic_conditions/adherence/en.

WHO (2003), *Adherence to Long-term Therapies: Evidence for Action*, World Health Organization, available at: http://www.who.int/chronic_conditions/adherencereport/en/index.html.

CHAPTER 10

The Use of Interactive Communications Technology in Disease Management and Compliance/Persistence Programmes

Dr Bill Byrom and David Stein

In this chapter we consider the use of interactive communication technologies such as Interactive Voice Response (IVR),[1] interactive text messaging (Short Message Service or SMS text) and the Internet and e-mail in compliance programmes. Such technologies are often used in combination with human interactions via integrated call centres, but may also be used to administer an entire programme. Throughout this chapter, application areas are illustrated with published case studies.

We explore the value of these technology approaches in the collection of patient-reported outcomes data and find out how these data can become central to the execution of a compliance programme. We also consider how these technologies can be used to provide reminder messages and to deliver education and counselling to increase patients' involvement with their treatment.

1. For those unfamiliar with IVR, these systems use the telephone as an interface between the patient and a central computer. Messages and questions are delivered by playing recorded voice files, and patients can answer questions by entering numeric data or selecting response options by using the numbers on the telephone keypad.

First, we explore how these technologies have been used in clinical trials to collect patient self-report data and assess the value of such data in routine patient care.

THE USE OF INTERACTIVE COMMUNICATIONS TECHNOLOGIES IN CLINICAL TRIALS

Interactive Voice Response (IVR) systems, the Internet and interactive SMS have already been used in research studies and clinical trials to interact with patients. The Internet and IVR systems have been used to deliver patient qualification screeners for candidates responding to media campaigns for clinical trials (Stein and Byrom, 2005). Interactive SMS messages have been used to collect simple outcomes data from patients in phase IV clinical trials (Davis, 2004) . Most significantly, however, IVR systems have been used in clinical trials for over 15 years to collect patient-reported outcomes data (Corkrey and Parkinson, 2002). For example, the US Food and Drug Administration (US FDA) approval of eszoplicone (Lunesta, Sepracor) for insomnia was based on primary efficacy data collected using sleep diaries administered using an IVR system. In addition, the prescribing information for the estradiol/levonorgestrel transdermal system (Climara PRO, Berlex), a hormonal transdermal patch treatment for post-menopausal symptoms, includes patient-reported bleeding/spotting data collected using an IVR system during a one-year clinical trial. The benefits of using IVR in the collection of patient-reported data include enhanced data quality and integrity which is important in the regulatory acceptance of clinical trials data (Byrom, 2004). Sophisticated IVR diary systems include reminder messaging approaches to ensure ongoing compliance with the diary schedule to minimize missing study data. Reminders include outbound recorded messages or SMS text messages to the patient's telephone, e-mail alerts to patients, and fax and e-mail alerts to the investigational site to trigger human follow-up.

The types of patient-reported outcome collected using IVR vary considerably: simple symptom diaries, withdrawal symptom questionnaires, escape medication use records, QoL instruments, health economic questionnaires, and even diagnostic interviews and clinical assessments. For example, the Mental Health Screener (see Kobak *et al.*, 1997) is an IVR interview that screens for the most common mental disorders, including: major depression, major depression in partial remission, dysthymia, rule-out for bipolar disorder, generalized anxiety disorder, panic disorder, social phobia, obsessive compulsive disorder, bulimia (purging versus non-purging type), binge-eating disorder, alcohol abuse and dependence. The IVR adaptation of the Hamilton Rating Scale for Depression (HAM-D) interview delivers structured questions to enable an underlying algorithm to score disease severity against 17 different items. In fact, the IVR HAM-D has been accepted by the FDA as a primary endpoint in major depressive disorder outpatient studies in place of subjective patient assessments by clinicians (Byrom *et al.*, 2005).

THE VALUE OF PATIENT-REPORTED OUTCOMES INSTRUMENTS IN ROUTINE CARE

In addition to their use in clinical trials, patient-reported outcomes instruments have demonstrated considerable value in routine patient care. There are many published examples that have shown this, two of which are detailed below.

Home blood pressure monitoring in hypertension

Cappuccio *et al.* (2004) report a meta-analysis of 18 randomized, controlled trials to determine the effect of home blood pressure monitoring on blood pressure levels and the achievement of hypertension targets. This meta-analysis comprised 1359 hypertensive subjects allocated to home blood pressure monitoring and 1355 allocated to routine monitoring within the healthcare system – for example, blood pressure readings taken on a scheduled basis at outpatient clinics and primary care settings. The analysis showed not only that home monitoring was associated with both lower clinic-recorded systolic and diastolic blood pressures and lower mean blood pressure, but also that, overall, 10 per cent more patients achieved clinic-recorded blood pressure targets when using home blood pressure monitoring. Although these improvements were relatively modest in their own right, the analysis concluded that home monitoring may represent an important adjunct to treatment that is likely to contribute to a better outlook for cardiovascular events. The reason for improved outcomes with self-monitoring is likely to be due to patients' improved awareness of their condition and improvements due to drug treatment. This may result in increased motivation to maintain therapy and comply with a dosing regimen, thus improving overall effective health management. The involvement of patients in managing their own blood pressures, where possible, is highly motivating and provides a greater sense of sharing in the treatment and management of their condition.

QoL instruments in oncology

A number of studies have illustrated the value of using quality-of-life (QoL) questionnaires in routine oncology practice (Detmar *et al.*, 2000, 2002a, 2002b; Velikova *et al.*, 2002, 2004). In a randomized, controlled trial, Detmar *et al.* (2002a) explored the use of a health-related QoL instrument (the European Organization for Research and Treatment of Cancer QoL Questionnaire – Core 30: QLQ-C30) in patients undergoing palliative chemotherapy. Patients (n=217) who had received at least two cycles of chemotherapy were invited to participate and were randomized to either complete the CLQ-C30 group or the control group. Those assigned to the CLQ-C30 group were requested to complete the 30-item questionnaire in the waiting room prior to their appointment with the physician, after which the results were scored and graphed and provided to both patient and physician prior to their meeting.

The study found that the use of a QoL instrument in this way resulted in a significant increase in the frequency with which health-related QoL issues were discussed. This included discussion of issues that are less observable (such as social functioning) or of a more diffuse and long-term nature (such as fatigue) which are often left unaddressed by healthcare practitioners. As a result, physicians identified a greater percentage of patients with moderate to severe health problems compared to the control group. The use of the QLC-C30 was also associated with increased patient satisfaction in terms of the perceived level of emotional support received from their physician. All ten physicians and 87 per cent of the patients felt that the use of a QoL questionnaire facilitated communication and expressed an interest in its continued use.

Interestingly, a second study reported the value of using the same QoL questionnaire even when results were not fed back to the physician (Velikova *et al.*, 2004). In this study, which involved 28 oncologists and 286 cancer patients, subjects were assigned to one of three groups: an intervention group (QLC-C30 with feedback of results to the physician); an attention-control group (QLC-C30 without feedback of results to the physician); and a control group (no QoL instrument used in clinic before the patient–physician meeting). Using a second QoL instrument (FACT-G), the study found significant improvements in patient QoL amongst the intervention and attention-control groups, compared to patients not completing the QLC-C30 during their routine clinic visits (see Figure 10.1). Interestingly, this suggests that completion of the questionnaire itself may have effect on patient well-being regardless of whether results are fed back to physicians. However, improved emotional well-being was associated with feedback of data, as was more frequent discussion of chronic non-specific symptoms, without prolonging the patient–physician meeting.

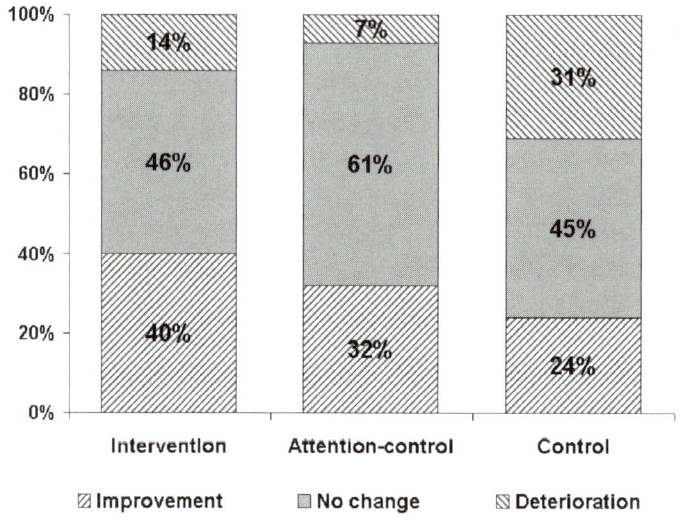

Figure 10.1 Proportions of patients showing clinically meaningful improvements, no change, or deterioration in FACT-G score after three encounters

In conclusion, patient-reported outcomes data collection can be of value in routine patient care. Their use is associated with enhanced patient–physician communication and can lead to improved patient outcomes even when data are not fed back to the physician. Involving patients in the routine collection of progress data increases their awareness and involvement in their treatment which may also result in enhanced outcomes due to better medication and treatment compliance.

The remainder of this chapter explores how technology solutions, such as IVR, SMS and e-mail, can be used to collect patient-reported outcomes data, and provide educational messages and counselling within disease management and compliance/persistence programmes.

FEATURES OF AN INTERACTIVE TECHNOLOGY SOLUTION FOR COMPLIANCE/PERSISTENCE PROGRAMMES

This section will focus on the use of interactive technologies in delivering, or providing a component of, disease management programmes. Although not an essential requirement, the collection of patient-reported outcomes can be a valuable component of such programmes.

The technologies we consider in this section are IVR, SMS and e-mail/Internet, and published case studies are used to illustrate their application. Interactions with these systems can be patient-initiated or computer-initiated. Before we explore the possible components of such a programme, we begin by considering the registration process.

Patient registration

One of the challenges in disease management is registering patients into a care programme. Although intended as a value-added service when associated with a particular treatment or therapy, this is unlikely to be the main driver affecting a physician's prescribing decisions. However, it is the point of prescription (that is, the physician's office) that provides the greatest opportunity for patients to be informed about, and to opt into, a compliance programme. In most cases, therefore, it is at the physician meeting where a programme associated with a particular drug is discussed, and the patient is given appropriate information to enrol on the programme should he or she desire to do so. Pharmaceutical medical representatives may be responsible for enrolling doctors within their territories into the programme. Interestingly, another significant healthcare touch-point that may be currently underutilized is the patient–pharmacist meeting at the point of medication dispensation. It is possible for programme details to be provided with the dispensed medication, or for a pharmacist to discuss a programme with a patient at the pharmacy. Many modern prescription and reimbursement systems provide the facility to remind pharmacists to deliver specific messages with certain dispensed medications, and they may receive remuneration for this.

Once informed about a programme, patients may formally enrol in a variety of ways: by mailing an enrolment card, registering via the Internet, or telephoning a toll-free number (see Figure 10.2). Although registration can be performed by an automated system, such as via a web page, there are advantages in providing a human interaction at this point. Therefore, the registration event will often be completed between the patient and a human operator, either as an inbound toll-free call made by the patient or as an outbound call made to the patient in response to registration via a mailing card or the programme website. The intention is to collect/confirm all contact details and capture background information essential in tailoring the programme to the individual needs of the patient. The registration process may also represent an important opportunity to reinforce the patient's health literacy (see box) by explaining key details related to the condition or treatment. In general, registration may include identification of:

- treatment targets and goals, such as weekly weight loss goals within an obesity programme
- patient risk category, which may be used in determining the content and nature of follow-up activities
- treatment expectations and concerns.

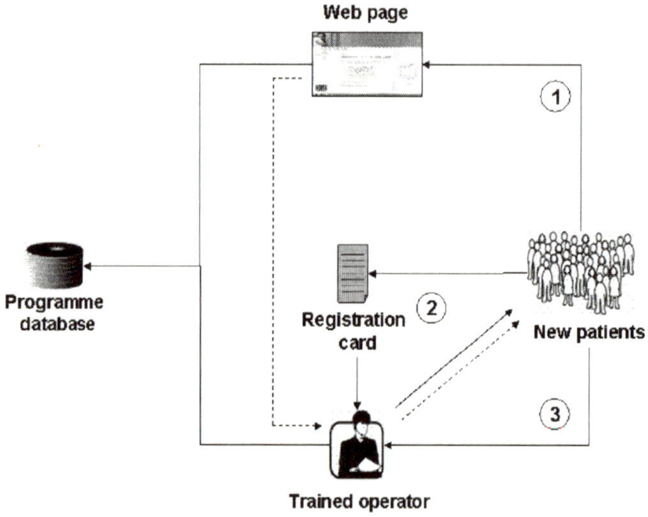

Figure 10.2 Programme registration via (1) web page access (which may include operator call-back), (2) registration card or (3) toll-free call

As part of their registration, online databases of participating doctors can be used to quickly establish the patients' physicians and clinic addresses. In addition, the following can be collected and transferred to the central computer that controls automated interactions:

- the patient's preferred method of contact: IVR, SMS, email or toll-free number
- the patient's phone number, mobile number or e-mail address (as appropriate)
- for outbound IVR reminders, the patient's preferred contact time (for example, 7–9 p.m.).

Patient reminders

Communications technologies such as e-mail, SMS and outbound recorded telephone messages have been successfully employed to deliver reminders to patients in routine care settings. In a disease management or compliance programme these messages might, for example, serve to remind the patient to take the medication as scheduled or to obtain a repeat prescription at the appropriate time. Making these messages interactive (see Figure 10.3) enables not just the message itself to be delivered, but also the collection of some simple feedback in order to tailor the programme to the patient's individual needs or behaviour, such as:

Health Literacy

Health literacy is an important concept for disease management programmes. The term is defined as: 'The degree to which individuals have the capacity to obtain, process, and understand basic health information and services needed to make appropriate health decisions' (US Department of Health and Human Services, 2000). One study of 979 emergency-room patients reported that 81 per cent had inadequate health literacy rates (Baker *et al.*, 1997). The healthcare industry consistently reports that this problem affects 90 million Americans. Such individuals may have significant difficulty understanding instructions from their doctor or pharmacist relating to their course of treatment. They may not understand the implications of failing to adhere to a dosing schedule or, for that matter, continuing to take their prescription medications. This is particularly challenging for preventive medications, such as those relating to Alzheimer's disease treatment, as when patients do not sense improvement they may stop taking their medications. The sad result is that their impairment continues unabated.

Health literacy also affects doctor–patient interactions. The *Wall Street Journal* reported that 80 per cent of patients forget most of their doctor's instructions immediately after an office visit. Also, half of what they think they remember is actually incorrect (Landro, 2003). Therefore, the use of interactive communications technologies for follow-up after an office visit has the potential to increase the patient's recall and understanding regarding treatment. Additionally, use of such communications prior to an office visit may facilitate more effective communication between the doctor and patient, as we shall see later in this chapter.

- intention to obtain a repeat prescription
- difficulties with the treatment or regimen
- satisfaction with the treatment compared to previous treatments
- effectiveness of the treatment
- health outcome data
- impact of disease on lifestyle/simple measures of quality of life.

For example, an IVR reminder scheduled around repeat dispensing dates may contain a message such as:

'Hello. This is your hypertension programme reminder call. Our information suggests that your current tablets should require replacing soon. Have you recently, or are you intending to, obtain a repeat prescription for drug X from your doctor? For "yes", press 1. For "no", press 2.'

'Over the last month, have you been satisfied with your blood pressure control using drug X? For "yes", press 1. For "no", press 2.'

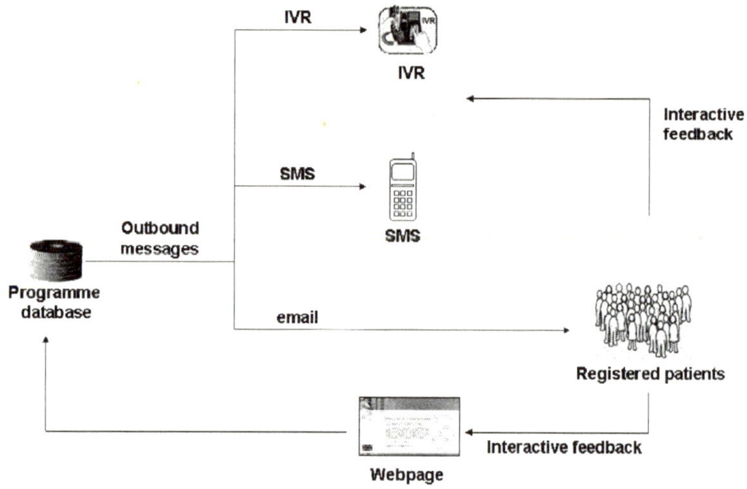

Figure 10.3 Outbound patient reminders and collection of interactive feedback using IVR, SMS and e-mail

Patients answering 'no' to any of the above questions might trigger additional follow-up such as literature fulfilment or even contact by a human operator.

An analogous interactive reminder message using SMS will consist of three messages (two outbound to the patient and one reply sent by the patient to the central computer) – for example:

> *'Hello [patient's name]. This is your drug X reminder. Reply back with "1" if you have/will obtain a new prescription or "2" if you intend to stop using drug X. Thank you.'*
> [Patient's reply]
>
> *'Thank you* [patient's name]. *We are pleased that you will continue with drug X.'*

E-mail reminders, as a third option for a patient, can operate in two ways. First, in a similar way to SMS, patients can reply to a received email message with a response. Following receipt of their response a 'thank you' email can be issued. Alternatively, an e-mail can contain links to a secure website at which feedback can be entered. The choice of solution will depend on the quantity of information to be collected, but generally it is anticipated that only small amounts of focused feedback will be collected during a reminder message.

At first, these kinds of interaction might be considered intrusive, particularly in the light of similar automated messaging employed within the telesales industry. However, in compliance programmes, it should be remembered that patients choose for themselves whether they wish to be contacted in this way and do so out of a desire to achieve important health outcomes and personal treatment goals. Published studies, in fact, present many examples of the successful utilization of communications technology to provide patient medication and appointment compliance reminders. Krishna *et al.* (2002) review the use of outbound recorded messages in 19 clinical studies, including paediatric and adult studies ranging from 16 to 3158 subjects. They conclude that automated telephone messages are successful in increasing compliance amongst patients and caregivers and in improving health outcomes. SMS has successfully been used in appropriate countries and populations. Dr David Green (2003) constructed an SMS reminder system to enhance medication compliance amongst patients suffering from tuberculosis (TB) in Cape Town, South Africa. TB treatment requires adherence to a strict regimen, usually four tablets five times a week for six months. Poor adherence to treatment regimens results in a low cure rate and an increasing incidence of multi-drug resistant strains of the TB organism. Interestingly, despite the socioeconomic background of the local population, over 50 per cent of people in the Cape Peninsula, and 71 per cent of TB patients at the clinic studied had access to a mobile phone. Dr Green's application issued SMS messages on a regular basis to over 300 patients, reminding them to take their medication. Of the 300-plus patients involved in the pilot study there were only five treatment failures, an outcome so successful that the scheme has been identified by the World Health Organization as an example of best practice. Interestingly, when his study commenced, patients complained to Dr Green that the message sent – 'Take your Rifafour now' – was too bland and boring. As a response, the system was changed to include jokes, pearls of wisdom and tips about lifestyle management in addition to a reminder to take medication. This fun element served to keep patients engaged with the messages and was more effective in providing the intended reminder. This finding is echoed by a similar pilot study of SMS reminders amongst young asthmatics in Scotland (Neville *et al.*, 2002). This study used a virtual friend, 'Max', who provided daily medication reminders. Study participants commended the researchers on the use of novelty lifestyle messages, and many even developed a rapport with their virtual friend and frequently sent messages back to 'Max'. Examples of some of the text message dialogues reported include:

'Bonjour, c'est Max. Hav U taken Ur inhaler yet?'
'Yea, I'm off to take it now.'

'Buenas noches. Max here. Forgotten something 2day?'
'Beat U 2 it. Just tkn it!'

'Yo dude, its Max reminding U2 take ur inhaler.'
'Yep dis morning.'

Although only a small pilot study in 30 patients, feedback suggested that the reminder system may have favourably influenced medication compliance. One patient reported that they regularly used to forget to take their inhaler two or three times each week but didn't miss any applications over the one-month pilot study period.

Although potentially less immediate than outbound IVR and SMS messaging, e-mail reminders have also been shown to be effective in improving medication compliance amongst patients with private e-mail accounts. A US study of 50 new oral contraceptive pill (OCP) users showed increased compliance as a result of daily e-mail medication reminders (Fox *et al.*, 2003). Reminders were issued automatically at around 8:30 a.m. (± 30 minutes) every day to subjects for three cycles of OCP use. Subjects were instructed to check their e-mails daily and reply to the reminder to confirm receipt. They were also instructed not to reply to the e-mail reminder with any medical concerns or questions as these may not be read. Instead, the clinic contact information was provided. Subjects were contacted by telephone if they did not reply to the e-mail reminders for more than one week. To assess OCP compliance, subjects completed a diary recording their OCP use. No pregnancies occurred during the study. Medication compliance, as measured by the daily diary records, indicated that OCP compliance was improved over rates reported elsewhere in the literature. The researchers quoted that, typically, around 20–50 per cent of OCP users occasionally miss pills, compared to the 10–28 per cent of subjects in their study who received daily e-mail reminders who missed pills. Overall most subjects reported that they found the e-mail reminders very helpful (19 per cent) or somewhat helpful (65 per cent).

Advice/motivational milestone messages

Outbound messages can also be used to provide timely advice of benefit to the patient. These can be individualized, based on other information known about the patient – for example, outcome status or main issues/concerns – or can be based around known longitudinal attitudes of the patient population as a whole.

A good illustrative example is reported in a research article exploring the reasons for non-compliance amongst patients treated with anti-depressants (Demyttenaere *et al.*, 2001). This study surveyed 272 patients, diagnosed with major depressive disorder and receiving anti-depressant therapy, using a compliance questionnaire. At the end of six months' treatment, 53 per cent of patients had discontinued anti-depressant treatment, a concerning number given that current treatment guidelines recommend at least six months' therapy for effective treatment. The most frequently cited reasons for dropping out were 'feeling better' (55 per cent) and adverse events (23 per cent). Interestingly, the authors broke down reasons for dropping out by length of time on treatment. Patients dropped out after an average of 6.5 weeks due to adverse events; because of 'lack of

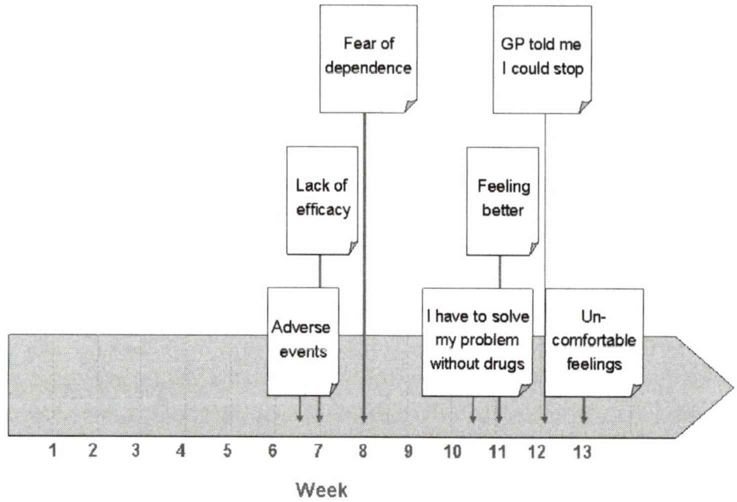

Figure 10.4 Reasons for ceasing anti-depressant treatment

efficacy' after 7 weeks; because of 'fear of drug dependence' after 8 weeks; and because 'I have to solve my problems without drugs' at 10.5 weeks. These and other reasons are presented in Figure 10.4.

This kind of information about patient non-compliance behaviour can be used to provide targeted information at the optimal time point during a compliance programme. For example, in the above situation, information about common side-effects and their persistence could be delivered at around week 6 so that patients feel well informed and have appropriate expectations when facing side-effects that might affect their medication treatment experience. Further, information about the importance of staying on treatment even when the patient feels much better and around the issue of dependence on anti-depressant treatments should (in this example) be delivered through weeks 8 to 11.

Information can be delivered through a variety of automated mechanisms, such as an outbound recorded message, which may be interactive to enable the patients to navigate quickly to find information about their most important issue, or e-mail, which may contain links to a programme web page containing useful in-depth information on the topics covered. Alternatively, an automated system may interact with a mail fulfilment facility which would be triggered to mail out information leaflets or packs on specified topics to specific subjects.

Collection and use of patient reported outcomes

As discussed previously, there is great value in the collection of patient-reported outcomes data as a component of a compliance or disease management programme. Not only does the collection of these data give patients greater self-involvement in their own care, but the data can also be used to tailor the programme and provide valuable naturalistic data to the sponsor.

Figure 10.5 illustrates how patients would normally interact with a system. As scheduled by the programme, patients would either call in to enter outcomes data via IVR or access a secure website to enter data online. Sophisticated systems would enable patients to use

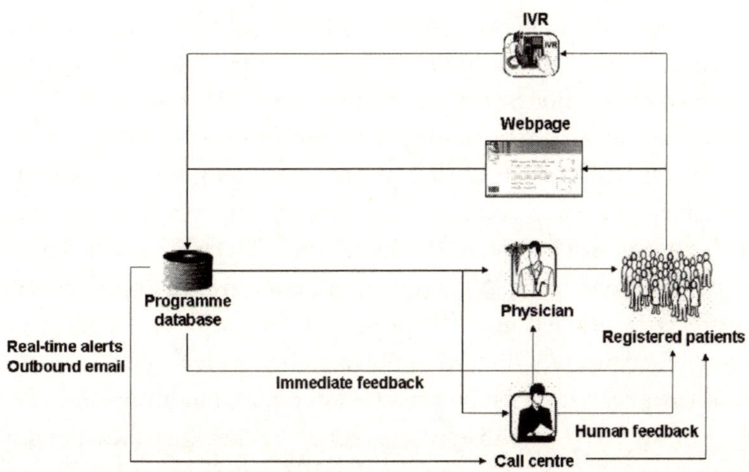

Figure 10.5 Patient-initiated collection of patient-reported outcomes data

either modality using the same username and password, and this flexibility may be important in patient uptake. Data entered are captured in a central database. The system itself can provide motivational feedback to the patient during the call or online session. For example, in an asthma programme, if the patient enters peak flow rates that remain in the target range, the system can inform the individual of this success, along with a measure of improvement since treatment commenced.

The database itself can trigger automated actions. For example, if a patient has been identified as moving into an at-risk group based on their outcomes data, this can create a real-time alert (sent by fax, e-mail or secure file transfer) to a call centre which can ensure that a qualified human operator will make a call to the patient. In the case when a call centre is also being used in combination with the technology, these outcomes data can also be fed back to the call centre on a regular basis so that they are available to supplement discussions should the patient call in or be contacted by a human operator. In addition, the outcomes data can be summarized into scheduled reports that are issued to the patient's physician.

Asking the patient to initiate these interactions is in itself a useful measure of motivation to participate in the programme. Patients who stop recording outcomes data may be losing the drive to continue with the programme, which may itself be as a result of issues or concerns with the medication. Identifying these patients early on enables additional follow-up, perhaps via a call-centre operator, where any concerns can be discussed and appropriate information provided.

This approach has proved successful in many applications. For example, Friedman *et al*, (1996) report a study evaluating the use of an IVR system within a programme of care for 267 hypertensive patients aged 60 years and over (mean age 76 years), which compared usual medical care with and without an IVR monitoring system. The IVR programme required subjects to call in on a weekly basis over a six-month treatment period. In addition to collection of outcomes (systolic and diastolic blood pressures), the IVR system also delivered questions regarding their understanding of their medication regimen (medication names, dosages and frequency of administration), their adherence to the regimen and whether or not they were experiencing any known side-effects. The system was designed to emulate the monitoring and counselling strategies and conversational style of a clinician and typically took around four minutes per call. Overall, medication adherence increased more amongst the patients receiving IVR monitoring (17.7 per cent versus 11.7 per cent) as measured by home pill counts performed by field technicians (Figure 10.6a). Significantly, adherence was greatly increased amongst those patients defined as non-adherent prior to commencing the study (taking < 80 per cent of their prescribed medication at baseline audit). In this subset, adherence increased by 36 per cent amongst the patients receiving the IVR programme, compared to 26per cent amongst routine care patients. In addition, the IVR programme was associated with greater improvements in blood pressure (Figure 10.6b). Amongst patients who were defined as non-adherent at baseline, systolic blood pressure was reduced by an average of 12.8 mm Hg with IVR compared to 0.9 mm Hg with routine care. Diastolic blood pressure reduced by an average of 6.0 mm Hg amongst the IVR programme patients compared to an increase of 2.8 mm Hg observed amongst those under routine care.

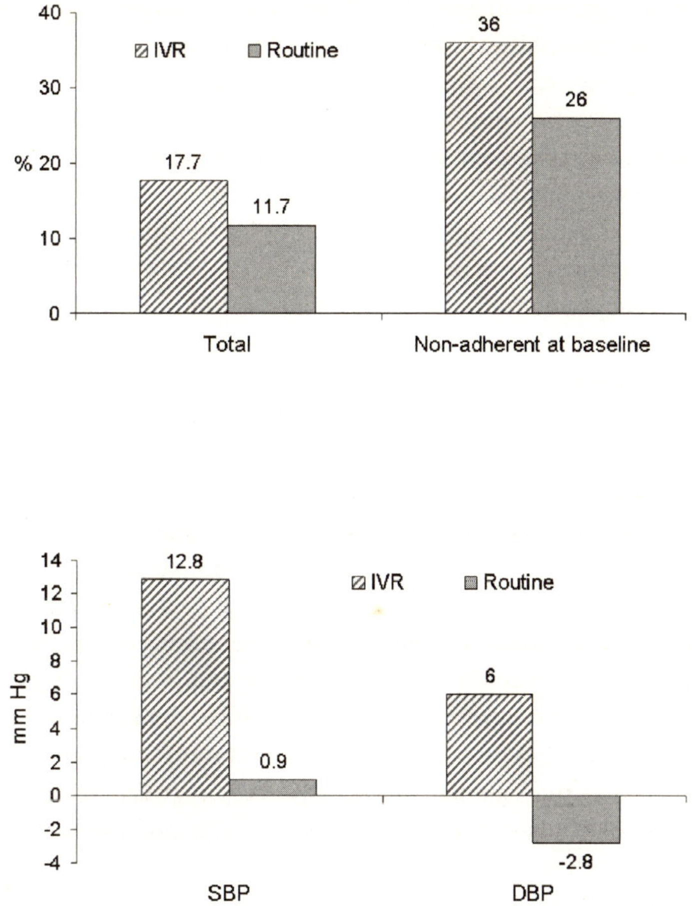

Figure 10.6 Improvements in (a) medication adherence and (b) systolic and diastolic blood pressures amongst patients receiving an IVR disease management programme compared to those receiving routine care

Patient satisfaction with this programme was high. When assessed using a 100mm visual analogue scale, 69 per cent of patients rated their satisfaction in the upper quartile of the scale and 54 per cent applied a similar rating when asked about the health benefits of the programme. Of the 102 physicians participating regularly, 85 per cent referred to the IVR reports. The study concluded that the improved blood pressure outcomes observed on the programme were a result of the increased medication adherence it produced. Another possible reason for these improvements, though not mentioned by the researchers, could be the enhanced patient care made possible by the outcomes data that were fed back to the physician. This information is of great value in facilitating medication adjustments or influencing counselling practice.

Triggered messages

An automated system can use the data collected to trigger messages to the patient. These can be via outbound call, e-mail, SMS, human operator call or mailing of literature.

When collecting patient outcomes data, these messages can be triggered when specific patterns of data are received, such as:

- deterioration of outcomes data
- reduced measures of patient satisfaction with treatment
- low self-reported medication adherence
- patient reports that the repeat prescription will not be obtained
- low QoL measures in specific domains
- adverse event profile.

These messages are triggered based on the patient profile and enable programmes to be individualized by timely interaction regarding current issues affecting the patient.

Messages are also recommended in cases where a patient fails to call in or visit the web page to record outcomes data for a sustained period of time. A simple reminder card or human operator call can be effective in returning them to the programme. In such cases, however, the reason for stopping recording outcomes may be some element of dissatisfaction with treatment. Perhaps they are experiencing adverse events, are disappointed with the treatment's efficacy, feel better and feel they don't need to continue with treatment, or are concerned about taking drug treatment for a sustained period of time. These concerns can be addressed by timely discussion with the patient, and appropriate literature; and the non-compliance with patient diary data recording can be an important indicator that these discussions are required before the patient ceases treatment and drops out of the programme.

Counselling/behavioural therapy

Automated approaches have been successfully used to deliver patient education and counselling – for example, in programmes for hypertension (Neville *et al.*, 2002), nutrition and exercise (Green, 2003; Glanz *et al.*, 2003) and smoking cessation (Ramelson *et al.*, 1999). These approaches use 'conversations' to question users, comment on their responses and deliver educational information or counselling in relation to targeted health behaviours. The Internet facilitates this kind of interaction and information delivery, but sophisticated IVR systems also provide a suitable vehicle for such programmes, often in combination with nurse or operator follow-up. Perhaps most practically, such an approach would work in combination with other information delivery media, particularly the direct mail of supporting literature. For example, based on the response profile of a patient during an IVR conversation, simple feedback can be delivered during the telephone interaction and followed up with a targeted mailing, the subject of which is prioritized from the patient data collected.

For example, Ramelson *et al.* (1999) developed an IVR system to counsel, educate and support patients attempting to give up smoking. The programme used an expert system to deliver automated dialogues that branched off down different pathways depending on patient responses. Dialogue was developed based on known psychological processes and behavioural models relevant to smoking cessation. Patients using the system were questioned and responded to each question by selecting an answer from a list of possible responses. The expert system could provide feedback to each possible response, and, based on the responses to a number of questions, additional information could be delivered comprising further feedback, counselling or even injecting humour into the encounter.

Powerful applications of such systems include the ability to individualize the programme to the immediate needs of the patient. This can be illustrated by the smoking cessation system. The application logic commences a patient encounter by determining their stage of smoking cessation, such as contemplating giving up, preparing to quit, actively given up for less than six months, maintenance and relapse phases. This analysis is then used to drive the direction of the subsequent conversation.

For example, if a patient is in the phase of contemplating giving up smoking, the system will assess the number of cigarettes smoked and provide feedback based on the change in number smoked since the last conversation with that patient. The system will identify reasons why the patient continues to smoke and reasons for wanting to quit and use this information to identify and review strategies to aid smoking cessation. When money is identified as a key driver for that individual, a dialogue such as that detailed below can be delivered:

'The money you spend on cigarettes adds up to a lot. Since you started smoking, approximately how many cigarettes on an average would you say that you have smoked?'
'30.'

'Approximately how many years have you been smoking?'
'25.'

'Do you realize that over the time that you have smoked, you have spent about US$27,375 on cigarettes? I'll bet you wish you had that money now. Well, it's not too late to quit smoking and save money now. If you continue to smoke for the next 10 years, you will spend another US$16,425 on your habit…' (Taken from Ramelson *et al.*, 1999)

This example illustrates another important consideration for successful disease management programmes – identification of the individual's treatment goals. These may in fact be unrelated to health outcomes – in this case, saving money to perhaps increase the standard of living or covering the expense of a holiday or new car. The identification of these individual goals and the provision of strategies to achieve them are, however, of great importance to the success of a full disease management programme.

Many of the programmes used in patient compliance and persistence utilize similar principles, although often in a simpler way. For example, feedback on health outcomes, medication compliance or adverse events can be used to provide tailored feedback and educational messages linked with targeted literature deployment. Knowledge of the profile of treatment adherence behaviour, and teasing out individual patient issues, enables the messaging to be tailored to a patient's specific needs.

Data reporting

In addition to direct feedback delivered during an interactive communication, such as a statement of progress relative to target in a programme in which hypertensive patients self-monitor their blood pressure, compliance programmes can also provide valuable reports to all key stakeholders.

Patients can receive reports detailing their progress with regard to health outcomes data collected or progress towards personal treatment goals, or even access such reports securely via the Internet. This provides valuable opportunities for patients to become more engaged with their treatment and, as a result, become more motivated in maintaining a treatment regimen. Such reports can also lead to patients not only seeing for themselves the benefit of self-assessment and maintaining treatment, but, when data are used to target communications and information deployment, it can also propagate a feeling that the programme is truly in tune and involved with their individual care.

As evidenced by some of the case studies reported earlier in this chapter, providing outcomes data to the caring physician is of benefit to both patient and physician. In such cases, outcomes data may, for example, be issued to the physician on a scheduled basis, perhaps once a quarter, in the form of a simple tabulated report created by the programme application. These data may provide valuable additional information that can contribute to decisions regarding the patient's care and enhance patient–physician interactions. There may, however, be additional reasons why programme data may be of value to physicians and which may also influence their decision to participate and offer the programme to patients under their care. New (2004–5) changes in the UK general practitioner (GP) contract, for example, contain targets regarding the care of patients in a number of key disease indications and therapy areas. GPs who achieve care targets are awarded points which translate into annual government funding for their practices. One such disease indication included in the contract is hypertension, and, to earn points, GPs need to demonstrate the achievement of target blood pressures amongst their patients. A compliance programme in hypertension might, therefore, include self-monitoring of blood pressures and the collection and reporting of these data in such a way as to assist the GP practice in demonstrating progress against national targets.

In addition to providing value to the treating physician, compliance and outcomes information is important to managed care organizations, healthcare insurers and other payers. These organizations have a vested interest in ensuring that patients adhere to their treatment, use their prescriptions properly and receive quality care from their doctors. It is not difficult to recognize the value of helping a patient to take a medication that will prevent costly hospital visits.

Finally, compliance programmes collecting health outcomes, QoL, compliance and patient satisfaction data provide a rich stream of information valuable in additional product marketing and public relations campaigns. Although sponsor companies may not obtain individual subject data, aggregated reports provide a rich picture of the treatment under naturalistic conditions. Such reports of data collected across a large population of patients may influence future prescribing attitudes. Subsets of data may also be reported on a regional level, providing medical sales representatives with useful relevant information to discuss in meetings with physicians and to use as a lever to see physicians who may otherwise be reluctant to devote time to a meeting.

PRACTICAL CONSIDERATIONS

When building a compliance programme application using interactive technologies, or with a component of these, there are a number of practical considerations that should be resolved. These are detailed below in the programme checklist (Table 10.1).

Experienced technology providers can advise on the resolution of many of these technical considerations with solutions tailored to a specific programme.

Table 10.1 Programme considerations checklist

Item	Detail
Withdrawal of consent to participate in programme	How the system should be updated to ensure contacts with withdrawn patients are terminated in a timely manner.
Patient authentication	Outbound SMS or e-mail interactions may be considered personal as these are issued to private mobile phone or e-mail accounts. Outbound IVR, however, may be answered by others using the same telephone number. In this case, it may be necessary to authenticate the patient prior to delivering a message. This may include issuing a pass code or using a birth date to authenticate the patient. Inbound communications by the patient using IVR will require patients to enter a pass code to reveal their identity and ensure that data are associated with previous data recorded by the patient.
Outbound messaging protocol	*Outbound email*: Successful delivery and opening of a message can be determined if required. Action to perform upon non-receipt or ignoring of the message should be considered, such as direct mail of a 'failure to reach' card. *Outbound SMS*: Actions to perform in the event of failed delivery or invalid mobile phone number should be determined, such as direct mail of a 'failure to reach' card. *Outbound IVR*: As above, actions to perform in the event of an invalid telephone number should be determined such as direct mail of a 'failure to reach' card. Additional considerations include: ● what time of day to call the patient ● how often and at what times should the system try to recall a patient if the telephone is engaged ● how often and at what times should the system try to recall a patient if the telephone is unanswered ● what to do if the system detects an answer machine.

Item	Detail
Change of contact preferences	Ability to change primary contact medium between IVR, SMS and e-mail.
Change of contact details	Ability to change contact addresses, e-mail and telephone details as required.
Data protection legislation	Ensure system and database procedures adhere to relevant data protection / HIPAA legislation.
Content of messages / interactions	Determining the content of messages with consideration of: ● overall programme objectives ● known key patient reasons for discontinuation ● common patient treatment goals ● properties and common side-effects of treatment ● recommended duration of treatment for successful health outcomes.
Length of messages/interactions	Determining the length of messages so that interactions remain valuable and motivating to the patient and not burdensome. Message length can be determined relative to the quantity of interaction, the value of feedback and educational messages and the frequency with which interactions are scheduled.
Frequency of messages/interactions	Determination of the optimal frequency of message delivery. This may not be uniform across a programme. For example, medication reminders may be issued daily for an initial period, and when satisfactory compliance is achieved the frequency may be reduced or reminders may be turned off completely. In addition, patient-reported outcomes might be reported weekly or as desired by the patient, and counselling messages may be increased during periods when patients face, or are likely to face, known issues and concerns with the medication.
Amount of message repetition	Reminder messages, in particular, may be quite repetitive in nature. Programmes should consider a variety of messages, including the use of humour, lifestyle tips and so on, to minimize any apparent repetition.
Balance of outbound and inbound interactions	It is normal that inbound interactions initiated by the patient are used for most events at which patient self-report measurements are collected, particularly if these involve use of external recording equipment such as a peak flow meter or blood pressure monitor. Many educational, reminder and milestone interactions can be outbound to the patient using a variety of IVR, SMS, e-mail and direct mail. Inbound interactions have the benefit of providing a measurement of patient engagement with the programme, which may indicate treatment issues or concerns if changes are observed.

Item	Detail
Balance of human and automated interactions	The balance between human and automated interaction should be determined. This may be different for different patient subgroups, as may the media of automated interactions. The degree of human interaction may also change at different points in the programme. For example, medication reminders may be delivered by a human operator initially, and then replaced by an automated approach once the patient has become comfortable with the programme. Alternatively, patients identified as experiencing important issues or reduced satisfaction with the medication regimen may warrant a period of increased human contact. It is important to consider what will be effective within the constraint of the target return on investment expected from the programme.
Details and value of patient reported data	Patient-reported outcomes should be incorporated when they can be of value to the patient in providing a realistic metric through which they can self-monitor their treatment. These may include symptom measures and simple QoL assessments to enable progress through time and maintenance of therapy to be observed.
Feedback to healthcare providers	Where physicians and patients agree, feedback reports to the patient's doctor can provide information valuable to the patient's ongoing care. Reporting frequency, format and medium should be carefully considered and agreed.

CONCLUSIONS

Interactive technologies can provide a valuable component of compliance and disease management programmes, and can be used independently or in combination with human operator interactions. In particular, the electronic collection of patient-reported outcomes using either gold standard or bespoke instruments and diaries provides a valuable opportunity for patients to become more engaged with their treatment and to obtain appropriate and motivational feedback on their progress. Where possible and appropriate, this feedback can provide useful insights to enhance the physician–patient meeting either by direct reporting of outcomes to the physician or by providing reports that patients can bring to their appointments. Much published work shows the value and success of these techniques in providing reminders, collecting outcomes and providing education and counselling.

This chapter also demonstrated that patient acceptance of these approaches is high. Patients find these approaches helpful when they are used to provide positive and useful benefits towards their health-related and personal goals.

Although this chapter has not focused on return on investment, this is an important consideration, and technology solutions present a highly cost-effective approach to disease management programmes.

Overall, the use of inbound and outbound automated calls, text messaging and e-mail provide valuable means of communicating directly with patients and delivering patient care programmes aimed at improving the individual's experience of a treatment, raising the level of health literacy and improving health outcomes, treatment compliance and loyalty.

REFERENCES

Baker, D.W., Parker, R.M., Williams, M.V., Clark, W.S. and Nurss, J. (1997), 'The Relationship of Patient Reading Ability to Self-Reported Health and Use of Health Services', *American Journal of Public Health*, **87**, pp. 1027–30.

Byrom B. (2004), 'Electronic Diary Solutions: Enhanced Collection of Patient Reported Outcomes Data', *European Business Review*, Autumn, pp. 90–94.

Byrom, B., Stein, D. and Greist, J. (2005), 'A Hotline to Better Data', *Good Clinical Practice Journal*, **12**(2), pp. 12–15.

Cappuccio, F.P., Kerry, S.M., Forbes, L. and Donald, A. (2004), 'Blood Pressure Control by Home Monitoring: Meta-analysis of Randomised Trials', *British Medical Journal*, **329**(7464), pp. 145–48.

Corkrey, R. and Parkinson, L. (2002), 'Interactive Voice Response: Review of Studies 1989–2000', *Behavior Research Methods, Instruments and Computers*, **34**(3), pp. 342–53.

Davis, T. (2004), 'Text to Win', European Pharmaceutical Executive, January–February, pp. 34–36.

Demyttenaere, K., Enzlin, P., Dewé, W., Boulanger, B., De Bie, J., De Troyer, W. and Mesters, P. (2001), 'Compliance with Antidepressants in a Primary Care Setting, 1: Beyond Lack of Efficacy and Adverse Events', *Journal of Clinical Psychiatry*, **62**, pp. 30–33.

Detmar, S.B., Aaronson, N.K., Wever, L.D.V., Muller. M. and Schornagel, J.H. (2000), 'How Are You Feeling? Who Wants to Know? Patients' and Oncologists' Preferences for Discussing Health-related QoL Issues', *Journal of Clinical Oncology*, **18**, pp. 3295–301.

Detmar, S.B., Muller, M.J., Schornagel, J.H., Wever, L.D.V. and Aaronson, N.K. (2002a), 'Health-related QoL Assessments and Patient–Physician Communication: A Randomised Controlled Trial', *Journal of the American Medical Association*, **288**, pp. 3027–34.

Detmar, S.B., Muller, M.J., Schornagel, J.H., Wever, L.D.V. and Aaronson, N.K. (2002b), 'Role of Health-related QoL in Palliative Chemotherapy Treatment Decisions', *Journal of Clinical Oncology*, **20**, pp. 1056–62.

Fox, M.C., Creinin, M.D., Murthy, A.S., Harwood, B. and Reid, L.M. (2003), 'Feasibility Study of the Use of a Daily Electronic Mail Reminder to Improve Oral Contraceptive Compliance', *Contraception*, **68**, pp. 365–71.

Friedman, R.H., Kazis, L.E., Jette, A., Smith, M.B., Stollerman, J., Torgerson, J. and Carey, K. (1996), 'A Telecommunications System for Monitoring and Counselling Patients with Hypertension: Impact on Medication Adherence and Blood Pressure Control', *American Journal of Hypertension*, **9**, pp. 285–92.

Glanz, K., Shigaki, D., Farzanfar, R., Pinto, B., Kaplan, B. and Friedman, R.H. (2003), 'Participant Reactions to a Computerised Telephone System for Nutrition and Exercise Counselling', *Patient Education and Counseling*, **49**, pp. 157–63.

Green, D. (2003), 'South Africa: A Novel Approach to Improving Adherence to TB Treatment', *Essential Drugs Monitor*, **33**, p. 8.

Kaplan, B., Farzanfar, R. and Friedman, R.H. (2003), 'Personal Relationships with an Intelligent Interactive Telephone Health Behaviour Advisor System: A Multimethod Study Using Surveys and Ethnographic Interviews', *International Journal of Medical Information*, **71**, pp. 33–41.

Kobak, K.A., Taylor, L., Dottl, S.L., Greist, J.H., Jefferson, J.W., Burroughs, D., Mantle, J.M., Katzelnick, D.J., Norton, R., Henk, H.J. and Serlin, R.C. (1997), 'A Computer-Administered Telephone Interview to Identify Mental Disorders', *Journal of the American Medical Association*, **278**(11), pp. 905–10.

Krishna, S., Balas, E.A., Boren, S.A. and Maglaveras, N. (2002), 'Patient Acceptance of Educational Voice Messages: A Review of Controlled Clinical Studies', *Methods of Information in Medicine*, **41**, pp. 360–69.

Landro, L. (2003), 'The Informed Patient', *Wall Street Journal*, 3 July.

Neville, R., Greene, A., McLeod, J., Tracy, A. and Surie, J. (2002), 'Mobile Phone Text Messaging Can Help Young People Manage Asthma', *British Medical Journal*, **325**, p. 600.

Ramelson, H.Z., Friedman, R.H., Ockene, J.K. (1999), 'An Automated Telephone-based Smoking Cessation Education and Counselling System', *Patient Education and Counseling*, **36**, pp. 131–44.

Stein, D. and Byrom, B. (2005), 'Meeting Patient Recruitment Timelines', *European Pharmaceutical Contractor*, Spring, pp. 56–58.

US Department of Health and Human Services (2000), *Healthy People 2010: Understanding and Improving Health* (2nd edn), Washington, DC: US Government Printing Office, November.

Velikova, G., Brown, J.M., Smith, A.B. and Selby, P.J. (2002), 'Computer-based QoL Questionnaires May Contribute to Doctor–Patient Interactions in Oncology', *British Journal of Cancer*, **86**, pp. 51–59.

Velikova, G., Booth, L., Smith, A.B., Brown, P.M., Lynch, P., Brown, J.M. and Selby, P.J. (2004), 'Measuring QoL in Routine Oncology Practice Improves Communication and Patient Well-being: A Randomised Controlled Trial', *Journal of Clinical Oncology*, **22**, pp. 714–24.

CHAPTER 11

Patient Compliance: Putting Interventions into Practice

Alan Blaskett

In healthcare, it is rare to achieve consensus across all stakeholder groups. However, on the matter of 'compliance with treatment', there is universal agreement across the medical profession, government, industry and, most importantly, patients: compliance rates must be addressed to achieve optimum health benefits, most appropriate use of limited healthcare resources and cost benefits for each nation's healthcare budget.

It is this consensus that perhaps offers the greatest opportunity to improve compliance rates. In isolation, each of the stakeholders has made little impact. However, in recent years, we have started to see some cooperative initiatives that have provided some positive signs for the future. While there remains much work to be done, with all stakeholders benefiting from the improved taking of medicines, there is good cause for optimism that government, medical professionals and industry can work in collaboration for the benefit of patients.

In this chapter, the role that the pharmaceutical industry is currently playing to complement the efforts of individuals, health professionals and the health services in the support of patients will be discussed and additional opportunities for cooperation between stakeholders explored.

THE NATURE OF POOR COMPLIANCE

Historically, it was the patient who was 'blamed' for poor compliance with treatment. Doctors wrote a prescription and provided instructions that patients were expected to follow, with poor rates of compliance often attributed to simple forgetfulness. We have grown to understand that the factors that influence compliance and treatment adherence are many and varied and that forgetfulness is not the primary cause as the majority of patients are able to articulate their reasoning for choosing to alter their dosage schedule or discontinue therapy.

In a group of patients who were monitored following the initiation of anti-depressant therapy only 10 per cent of those who had discontinued treatment after six months had done so under their doctor's instruction (see Figure 11.1).

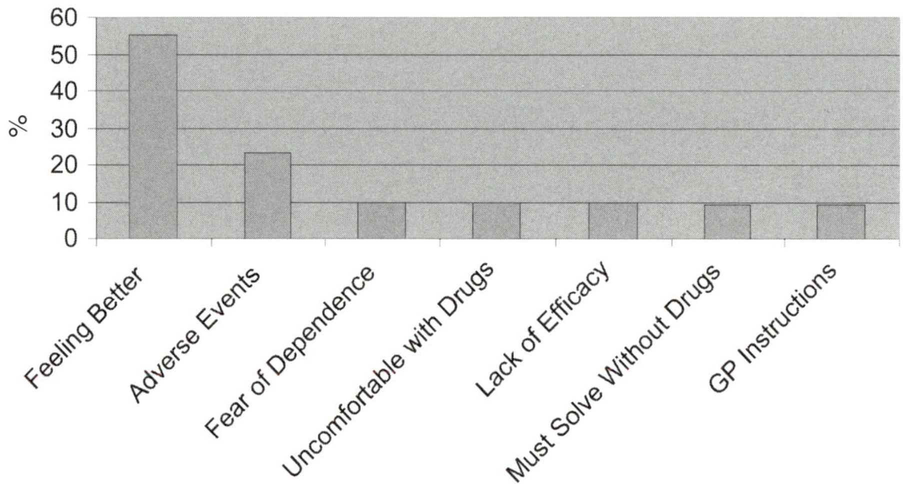

Source: Demyttenaere *et al.* (2001).

Figure 11.1 Reasons for discontinuing anti-depressant therapy

The study demonstrates that, rather than 'forgetting' their medication, patients made active decisions regarding their treatment without consulting their healthcare team.

With a lack of access to additional education or follow-up support, patients will make important decisions in isolation often based on unfounded beliefs, unrealistic expectations or misinformation. It therefore becomes critical that all stakeholders play their part in ensuring that, at a minimum, patients have access to sufficient resources to enable them to make well-informed decisions.

The World Health Organization report, *Adherence to Long-term Therapies: Evidence for Action* (2003) identifies five 'dimensions' that impact upon adherence with treatment:

- social/economic factors
- healthcare team and system-related factors
- condition-related factors
- therapy-related factors
- patient-related factors.

With no single intervention strategy proving to be effective for all patients and conditions, the report identifies that interventions need to be tailored specifically for the needs of the individual patient, demand a multidisciplinary approach and require follow-up due to the dynamic nature of adherence issues. Unfortunately, by their very nature, patient-tailored interventions are time-consuming and a heavy burden to implement within the already stretched resources of the existing health services.

Although it is now well acknowledged that compliance is a shared responsibility, in practice circumstances often limit the ability of the healthcare team to provide as much support to patients as they require. Despite best intentions, short consultation times, limited patient education resources and infrequent patient follow-up opportunities can result in few observable changes in the doctor–patient relationship.

WHAT IS INDUSTRY DOING TO HELP?

Increasing the effectiveness of adherence interventions may have a far greater impact on the health of the population than any improvement in specific medical treatments.
(WHO, 2003)

If the role of the pharmaceutical industry is to improve the health of patients through the development of ever more effective medicines, then ensuring that those therapies are taken to best effect must also be within the industry's responsibilities.

In 1995 the Royal Pharmaceutical Society of Great Britain, in partnership with Merck Sharp & Dohme, undertook an inquiry into the difficulties encountered by patients taking prescribed medicines. It concluded that patients' failure to take medicines to best effect could be damaging, and indeed devastating, for the individuals concerned and their families. For the National Health Service it constituted two forms of wastage: first, the minimization of the potential benefits of drug therapy; second, the extra cost of treating the avoidable consequent morbidity.

At the time of the study, it was concluded that problems arise because of the pervasive failure to establish effective therapeutic partnerships between doctors, other healthcare workers and their patients. The study offered the then radical view that the target should be to achieve 'concordance' – where patients are enabled to actively participate in treatment decisions – rather than 'compliance' with a doctor's instructions.

As a result of this work, the UK National Health Service has accepted the challenge to improve the communications between doctors and patients. A number of initiatives have been taken to highlight the need for increased participation of patients in their treatment decisions and improved access to appropriate medical information. The goal is to improve communications with patients, increase involvement in the treatment decision and gain greater patient understanding and commitment to prescribed therapy.

Industry is well positioned to cooperate with the health services in achieving these goals. There is mutual benefit in improving patients' understanding of, and commitment to, therapy while manufacturers also have the resources and expertise necessary to develop educational materials to be made available to patients through their healthcare team.

The pharmaceutical industry has been providing various resources to assist healthcare professionals in the care and education of patients for many years. It is important to recognize that, with these resources, the industry is focused on the support of existing patients as opposed to promoting medications for new patients. In the provision of these items, the industry has remained at arm's length from patients, making such resources available through the patient's healthcare team.

Educational materials have usually been developed specifically for those patients who have been recently prescribed a new medication and have employed a variety of media. Examples include:

- printed product information
- product 'starter kits' (often including a product sample)
- audio cassettes
- patient videos/DVDs.

While these educational materials are certainly of benefit in improving access to quality health information, they do not address the critical aspects of individual patient needs, multidisciplinary support or follow-up. The WHO *Adherence Report* confirms that information alone is insufficient to drive improved compliance, because a patient's individual needs must also be addressed. A more comprehensive, interactive approach is required to identify patient-related issues that affect compliance.

In more recent years, with increasing access to the Internet, the pharmaceutical industry has also made support materials and interactive tools available online for patients. With branded direct-to-consumer (DTC) advertising of prescription medicines illegal in practically all markets other than the United States, it remains important to differentiate between the general public and prescribed patients. Product-specific material may only be made available to patients who have already been prescribed and have requested that information. To ensure that such websites are not accused of DTC advertising, product-specific material can be password-protected and only accessible after patients have validated that they have been prescribed the product in question. In practice, health professionals continue to regulate the access to online support materials as the registration of patients is generally facilitated by a member of the healthcare team.

The pharmaceutical industry also has a history of providing additional human resources to support patients. In many countries, industry-sponsored specialist nurses have been made available to provide patient education and conduct clinics. Diabetes and multiple sclerosis are two therapeutic areas that have benefited from this practice in various countries. With the support of the healthcare team, industry-sponsored nurses provide non-promotional support, education and, in some cases, ongoing care to patients. The industry recognizes that well-educated, supported and motivated patients demonstrate improved compliance and achieve better health outcomes. Ensuring that patients are supported to use products most effectively is both ethical and good business practice. Patients benefit with improved support and health, the healthcare team benefits with access to additional resources and the pharmaceutical industry benefits with patients who are more likely to maintain therapy.

Unfortunately, the provision of industry-sponsored nurses is not practical for all conditions. Although sponsored nurses are an option for some specialist areas with relatively small patient populations, more widespread conditions would be impractical to support with such a scheme. For larger (or more remote) populations or conditions which require regular follow-up, specialist medical call centres are an emerging option that is increasingly being used, in a cooperative venture between industry and the medical profession, to provide professional nurse support to prescribed patients.

THE ROLE OF NURSE CALL CENTRES

Nurse call centres provide patients with reliable and efficient access to medical information from qualified health professionals. Patients benefit from the convenience of the enhanced access to support while the programme sponsor benefits from the efficiencies that are generated through the use of a call centre.

In the UK, NHS Direct has been established to provide the public with direct access to health information via the phone. Many patient enquiries can be resolved on the phone or, alternatively, patients can be directed appropriately within the NHS infrastructure, ensuring that limited resources are used most effectively.

Industry-sponsored nurse call centres generally provide patients with access to additional information and support specific to a particular medical condition or therapy. Such services are an extension of the educational support that the industry has provided to patients over the years. The same controls are applied to the information that is delivered during a discussion with a call-centre nurse. Information must continue to be:

- educational rather than promotional
- available only to those who request it
- supportive of the healthcare team's treatment decisions
- validated and within the bounds of approved product information.

However, as direct communication is established with patients, nurse call centres have additional responsibilities:

- Patients must be referred to their healthcare team as necessary.
- Privacy laws must be adhered to and patient confidentiality respected.
- Adverse events must be filed with the authorities.

The benefit for patients is clear. In line with the principles of 'concordance', with additional support and access to information, patients are empowered to take greater responsibility for their treatment. As phone calls permit more regular follow-up contact to be made, patients have increased involvement, and individual patient concerns can be addressed, ensuring that compliance and adherence to treatment is enhanced.

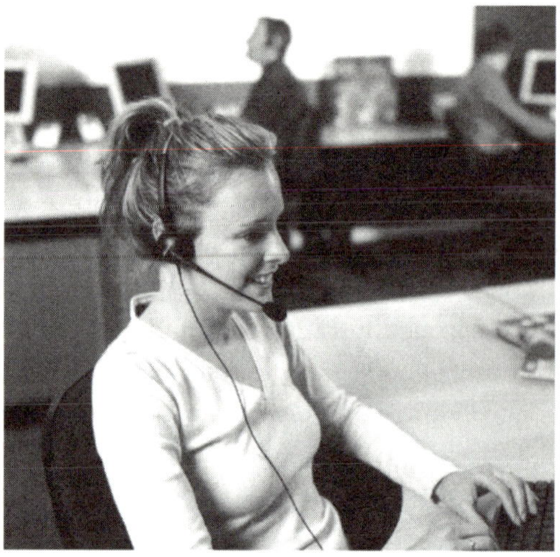

Figure 11.2 Nurse at work within the International SOS Patient Support Department, London

Invariably, the success of a telephone support programme depends on the cooperation of all stakeholders. Programme design, ethics approval, implementation and delivery require input from all parties.

As is often the practice with printed materials or the development of a patient-oriented website, programme design is a collaborative effort. In practice, the sponsoring company generally leads the process, consulting recognized medical experts for their input on content. As patients' needs are paramount, patient associations often contribute further insights into the patient's perspective.

In some countries formal approval by government authorities is required but, even in those where this is not mandatory, programmes are often presented to ethics committees prior to implementation. It is critical that programmes are designed to ensure that patient confidentiality is maintained, that patients are fully informed prior to choosing to participate and that the programme content is accurate, balanced and complementary to the support provided by the patient's healthcare team.

Further cooperation is required to ensure that support programmes are brought to the attention of patients and the opportunity to participate made available. With members of the healthcare team responsible for the facilitation of registration into programmes, even the most well-designed interventions will fail due to lack of participation without their support and endorsement of the service to be provided.

Although access to professional nursing staff on the phone can be of great comfort to patients and assist in ensuring the most appropriate use of healthcare resources, the limitations of telephone communication must be acknowledged. Throughout the duration of the programme, call-centre nurses refer patients back to the healthcare team as necessary. Programmes are most effective when positioned as an adjunct to the support of the existing healthcare team.

Ultimately, it is the participation and cooperation of the patients themselves that will determine the success of a compliance programme. Patients must be respected, listened to and have their needs addressed to ensure that they remain engaged with the programme and committed to their treatment. Should they fail to see any clear benefit of a programme they will soon withdraw and any opportunity to improve compliance will be lost.

Although nurse call centres are a relatively new tool to be applied in the management of compliance, examples of such programmes can be found across a wide range of therapeutic areas and countries. The following is a non-exhaustive list of conditions that are currently supported by nurse call centres in Europe, North America, South America, Asia, Australia and Africa:

- congestive heart failure
- diabetes
- hepatitis C
- hypertension
- multiple sclerosis
- obesity
- osteoporosis
- rheumatoid arthritis
- smoking cessation
- travel vaccination.

Despite the variations in regulations, healthcare environment and available technology between countries, it has been shown that opportunities exist to implement nurse call-centre programmes across all continents.

Provided that it is the patients' welfare that remains the primary objective of any programme, health professionals, health services and industry have an excellent opportunity to work together to develop innovative solutions that enhance service to patients, drive improved compliance and reduce the cost of healthcare.

CHALLENGES

Despite the precedent of phone-based compliance programmes to be found in the majority of pharmaceutical markets, there are a number of hurdles to overcome in the implementation of new programmes.

Published results

Perhaps the greatest barrier to the adoption of new programmes is the lack of published data proving the effectiveness of phone-based initiatives. Of the work that has been published, results have been positive but often limited to self-reported patient data or presented without a control group.

The lack of published evidence is due to a combination of factors:

- Nurse call centre programmes are still a relatively new innovation so there are a limited number of case studies to draw upon.
- Sponsors are reluctant to share details of their programmes.
- It is difficult to isolate a control group when the process of recruiting patients and monitoring results in itself is likely to have some impact on patients' commitment to therapy.

It is hoped that, with time, more programme sponsors will be willing to share their results. In the meantime, pioneers have proceeded on the basis of anecdotal feedback from patients and their healthcare team or observations of adherence rates of patients 'in market' versus those experienced during clinical trials. It is often the case that adherence rates during clinical trials are superior to those in an open market. This may well be explained by the requirement that patients actively agree to participate in trials and the additional observation generally involved. To a large extent, telephone compliance programmes replicate these aspects of a formal trial, providing sponsors with the confidence that compliance rates comparable to those achieved during clinical trials can be anticipated.

Perceptions of advertising

The advertising of pharmaceuticals is highly regulated and, in the majority of markets, limited to communications directly with the medical profession. Pharmaceutical companies may fear that educational programmes to prescribed patients could be perceived as DTC advertising.

There is a need for all parties to recognize the difference between educational programmes for prescribed patients and promotion to the general public. Regulations in many markets fail to differentiate the two adequately, leaving a 'grey area' that does not benefit any party. In this situation, the responsibility falls to the sponsoring company to ensure that all stakeholders are actively involved in the development of programmes and to demonstrate that improving health outcomes for patients is the primary objective.

Registration

One of the common challenges for compliance programmes is in the recruitment of patients. Without the ability to promote the availability of programmes due to advertising regulations, registration of patients is dependent on health professionals encouraging patients to participate.

The processes to be established to maximize registration are therefore critical. Health professionals need to be kept aware of the programme's benefits to patients and to be provided with simple registration processes that will not be a burden on their limited time.

The most successful registration campaigns provide a range of registration options through each of the members of the healthcare team: the physician, the nurse and the pharmacist.

CONCLUSION

Compliance and adherence to therapy are complex issues with no obvious 'one size fits all' solution available. It appears that actively involving patients in treatment decisions, empowering patients with access to medical information and providing ongoing monitoring all contribute to improved compliance and adherence rates. The challenge for health services, however, is to provide these enhanced levels of support cost-effectively.

In recent years, industry-sponsored compliance programmes have provided some indications that improvements in compliance rates can be achieved by using remote technologies to support patients. If the further potential of these initiatives is to be explored, greater cooperation between stakeholders, more sharing of outcomes by sponsors and a greater trust of industry motives is needed.

With public health at stake and improved compliance rates a common goal for all stakeholders, the outlook is optimistic, with more compliance programmes expected to be made available for the benefit of patients in the coming years.

REFERENCES

Demyttenaere, K., Enzlin, P., Dewé, W., Boulanger, B., De Brie, J., De Troyer, W. and Mesters, P. (2001), 'Compliance with Antidepressants in a Primary Care Setting, 1: Beyond Lack of Efficacy and Adverse Events', *Journal of Clinical Psychiatry*, **62**, pp. 30–33.

Haynes, R.B. (2001), 'Interventions for Helping Patients to Follow Prescriptions for Medications', *Cochrane Database of Systematic Reviews*, Issue 1.

WHO. (2003), *Adherence to Long-Term Therapies: Evidence for Action*, World Health Organization, available at: http://www.who.int/chronic_conditions/adherencereport/en/index.html.

Part 4
Achieving Compliance: Looking to the Future

The preceding chapters have focused on how to plan for success from the start. Critically in preceding chapters, the difference between compliance and concordance has been touched upon. As the previous authors have made clear, healthcare interventions can only be successful if the individual receiving that intervention wishes to accept that intervention. The final two chapters of this book look at a future in which healthcare delivery is truly patient-focused and collaborative.

CHAPTER 12

No Quick Fix: Shared Decision-making and Tailored Patient Support as the Route to More Effective Medicine-taking

Caroline Kelham, Joanne Shaw and Geraldine Mynors

WHY PATIENT INVOLVEMENT IS THE FUTURE

Background

Prescribed medicine is the most common form of medical intervention, accounting for almost 15 per cent of all health expenditure. Medicine use is also rising: the average person in England received 13.1 prescription items in 2003, a 40 per cent increase over the previous decade (Department of Health, 2003). Medical advances mean that diseases previously regarded as terminal, such as AIDS and some cancers, are becoming long-term conditions needing long-term treatment. Getting the most out of medicines is vital for maximizing therapeutic benefit and public health.

At the same time, many people experience difficulties in managing medicines, and problems with medicines account for a significant proportion of emergency hospital admissions. For example, adverse reactions are implicated in up to 17 per cent of hospital admissions (Department of Health, 2001). Many patients also report that their lives are dominated by medicine-taking and the associated unwanted side-effects (Carter and Taylor, 2003). When these problems prevent patients from getting the full benefit of their treatment it imposes a huge burden of avoidable ill-health and premature mortality on patients. It also burdens the health system with significant cost through wasted medicines, drug resistance and, more importantly, in dealing with preventable illness and complications.

What the evidence tells us

We know that non-compliance with prescribed medicine prevents many people from getting the most out of medicines. Non-compliance comes in many forms: depending on the disease area, as many as one in five patients fail to take the first step of collecting a prescription from the pharmacy. Many patients on short-term medications depart from recommended doses within a day or two of starting treatment. And many of those on longer-term medication may take a break from their medication or vary their dose depending on how they feel. A review of the evidence (Horne and Weinman, 1999) concluded that compliance overall is approximately 50 per cent but varies across different medication regimens, different illnesses and different treatment settings.

There are many reasons why people do not take their medicines as prescribed, and it is helpful to categorize these into intentional and unintentional barriers to effective medicine-taking.

Practical and logistical difficulties may play a part in unintentional non-compliance – getting to the pharmacy, opening the container and remembering the details of a

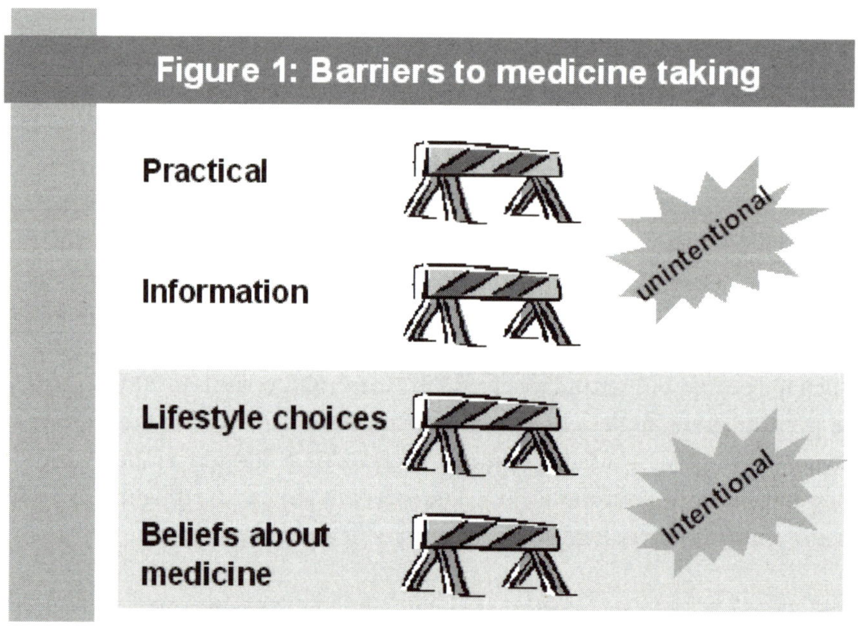

Figure 12.1 Barriers to medicine-taking

complicated regimen. However most non-compliance is intentional and results from conscious choices. Research shows that the most important factor determining whether, when and how patients take medicine, is their beliefs about the medication (Horne and Weinman, 1999).

The fact is that patients are not the passive recipients of prescribing decisions. They have their own views about medicines, how they should be used and how medicine-taking fits in with their daily lives. These views are based on a personal set of beliefs and understanding influenced by factors including the experience of family and friends, culture, education and social circumstances. They may be based on an incomplete understanding of the nature of the illness and the proposed treatment or at odds with scientific evidence. In other cases they may be based on a patient's own experience of medicine-taking and their knowledge about what fits in with their lifestyle.

Patients may be unsure from the start whether the benefit of taking medicine will outweigh the risks. In a poll conducted by MORI (2004) for 'Ask About Medicines Week', 30 per cent of the respondents said that they believed the risks of medicines are equal to, or greater than, the benefits. Some of these respondents had general concerns about what they see as the unnatural nature of medicines:

> *At one stage I was referred to a reflexologist, she was someone to talk to and was influential at that stage. She believed medication was a poison to the system so I came off the medication.*
> (Man, 61, Carter and Taylor, 2003)

Changes in society also mean that information, and particularly misinformation, about health and medicines is everywhere, of very variable quality. Drug scares highlighting the risks of certain types of medicine are common: recent examples have been hormone replacement therapy (HRT), the Pill (combined oral contraceptive pill) and the MMR (mumps, measles and rubella) vaccine. These often lead to unnecessary fears, negative consequences for patients and additional burdens on healthcare professionals. For example, a recent contraceptive pill scare in the UK about the risk of thrombosis led to a decrease in the overall use of oral contraceptives. It is estimated that terminations could have risen by up to 10 per cent as a result (Dillner, 1996), whilst there was in fact no significant difference in the incidence of venous thromboembolism in the period following the scare (Farmer *et al.*, 2000). The general public and individual patients need to develop a more realistic understanding of the risks and benefits of medicines and this will only happen when health professionals enter into more open and mature dialogue with patients about treatment choices.

Some patients also have strong beliefs about dependency:

> *I've got quite bad asthma but I always used to try to keep my inhaler use to a minimum. You don't want to be dependent on it. But then a nurse explained to me that I shouldn't feel bad about keeping my symptoms under control. It's made me feel much better about taking it and my health has really improved.*
> (Woman in her 30s, Carter and Taylor, 2003)

Others have general beliefs that have been influenced by family and friends:

> *I'm a devil for not taking tablets if I'm not careful, I have an in-built resistance to taking them. It stems from my mother as she would always say pills don't do you any good. I have changed my attitude now, but as soon as I can knock the drugs off I do … I don't like drugs but if someone convinces me I'll take them.*
> (Man, recovering from triple bypass, ibid.)

And others may not be convinced about the need for a particular medication or its efficacy:

> *You may think that the seizures have gone away so you don't need the medication. That may be right or it may be that the seizures have abated because you are taking medication.*
> (Woman, 40, ibid.)

> *It is a medication that does not make you feel better and if people can't actually see it is making them better, they may not continue.*
> (Nurse – National Osteoporosis Society, ibid.)

All these different sorts of belief play a very important role in a patient's conscious choice whether to take a medicine, reached as a result of weighing up perceived risks and benefits. Health professionals often know very little about these beliefs and make assumptions about what is 'best' for a patient that are very different from patients' own perceptions:

> *I should make it clear that I might be willing to shorten my life if it improved my quality of life. Doctors should be honest. They should talk about what it would mean to me and how I live my life … If you are in so much pain that you cannot move it may not be apparent to the doctor in his little kingdom.*
> (Levenson, 2002)

Research, surveys and people's individual stories show us that patients are making conscious decisions about whether to take medicines, based on their views, beliefs and experiences. People are therefore more likely to benefit from therapy when they understand the diagnosis and treatment, have had a chance to discuss their views and beliefs and are actively involved in decisions about the management of their condition.

Where does this lead us?

In the past, efforts to improve compliance have focused on providing clearer education and instruction about medicines, both written and face-to-face. Success in the future will involve looking at the problem of compliance from patients' perspectives: they are, after all, the ones taking the medicines and, in most cases, making decisions about medicine-taking. It is increasingly recognized that the key to making better use of medicines is involving patients as partners in decisions about their medicines – sometimes described as 'concordance'. Concordance is a new way for prescribers and patients to agree about medicines together. It looks for an alliance to be struck between prescribers and patients –

an agreement on how medicines will be used to solve the problem under discussion, after both of them have had their say.

This approach recognizes that the decision whether or not to take a medicine ultimately lies with the patient. A successful prescribing process will be an agreement that builds on the patient's experiences, beliefs and wishes to decide whether, when, how and why to take medicines. This agreement may not always be easy to reach, but without exploring and addressing these issues patients may not be able to get full benefit from the diagnosis and treatment of the illness.

It is important to note that concordance is not a new politically correct way of referring to compliance. Compliance measures patient behaviour: the extent to which patients take medicines according to the prescribed instructions. However, concordance measures a two-way consultation process: shared decision-making about medicines between a healthcare professional and a patient, based on a partnership in which the patient's expertise and beliefs are fully valued

Concordance, if achieved, may result in a different outcome from the consultation – for example, fewer medicines being prescribed than a doctor might initially think were 'optimal'. However, the medicines that are prescribed as part of a concordant agreement are more likely to be taken. There are also other important benefits in terms of safety. Patients who understand their drug treatment are better placed to pick up on prescribing, dispensing or administration errors.

OUR VISION OF THE FUTURE

Just as it is not a fashionable new word for compliance, neither is concordance a purely academic theory: work has been underway to identify practical ways of making it happen. The Medicines Partnership was set up by the UK Department of Health in 2002 to explore ways of putting a shared decision-making approach into practice. We have developed a model of what is required, comprising four essential components. This model is based on what patients tell us about their experiences and preferences, lessons from academic research and what we have learnt from our own experience of putting shared decision-making into practice through a national programme of work.

Patients have enough knowledge to participate as partners

- Patients have access to information about their condition, the treatment options available and the risks and benefits of different options relative to their own situation.
- Education empowers patients to manage their own health.
- Patients feel confident in asking questions and engaging in a discussion about medicines.

Health professionals are prepared for partnership

- Health professionals are equipped with the necessary skills to engage and share decisions with patients.

- Health professionals recognize that patients are decision-makers when it comes to medicine-taking.
- Health professionals invest time in reaching an informed agreement when necessary.

Prescribing consultations involve patients as partners

- Patients are invited to talk about medicine-taking.
- Professionals explain the treatment options.
- Patients are as involved as they want to be in treatment decisions.
- Patients and health professionals reach a shared agreement about the treatment to be followed.
- Patients' ability to follow treatment is checked.

Patients are supported in taking medicines

- Proactive support is offered to patients taking medicines.
- Medications are reviewed regularly with patients.
- All opportunities are used to discuss medicines and medicine-taking.
- Practical difficulties in taking medicines are addressed.
- Information is effectively shared between professionals.

Patients have enough knowledge to participate as partners

If patients are to participate in treatment decisions in a meaningful way, they need information. Many patients say that they do not have enough information about the options open to them, or the pros and cons of particular treatments. A public opinion survey carried out in the UK in 2004 (MORI, 2004) revealed that 44 per cent of people who had been prescribed a new medicine over the previous year felt that they did not know enough about other possible medicines or treatments. One in five felt they did not know enough about potential side-effects, and one in three said that there is not enough information available about the risks and benefits of medicines.

This is backed up by evidence from a recent international study where half of UK patients said that their doctor told them about treatment choices and asked for their ideas and opinions only occasionally or not at all (Schoen *et al.*, 2004).

Whilst health professionals may be concerned that telling people about side-effects might put them off taking medicines, what patients tell us from their own perspective suggests that the opposite may be true. A clear message coming though from patients is that having a better idea about what to expect, how long side-effects might last and what to do about them can help them make more informed judgements about medicine-taking.

> *If people were given more information they'd be more likely to take the medication, if there is a positive approach for example, 'these are the things to look out for, and if you have a problem come back to me'... The doctor and nurse did not tell me about side effects, but when I went back and said that I have problems like I need to scratch myself all over, then they told me.*
> (Man, 39 with depression and schizophrenia, Carter and Taylor, 2003)

There is not enough information, especially about side effects. They think: OK maybe if I don't take the medication for a couple of days the side effects will go away.
(Man, 58, ibid.)

If people experience problems but are not aware that there are any other options, this can also result in non-compliance:

I have had side effects and have gone back to the doctor. I needed to feel in control of my medication. I have had double vision, dizziness, loss of appetite, things like that. Some people with epilepsy have those side effects and don't realise that a change of dose or a change of medication can be helpful.
(Woman, 40, ibid.)

What kinds of information are patients looking for? It is clear that they value a range of sources: 82 per cent of respondents in our survey agreed that a range of types and source of medicines information is valuable. Health professionals are still seen as the main source of information with 69 per cent finding their doctor a useful source of information and 52 per cent going to their pharmacist (MORI, 2004).

I had a heart attack in 1998 and after that I did a cardiac rehab course. We had talks from the pharmacist and that was really helpful, telling us things we wouldn't have known ... also, he explained about when to take the medication, what time of day, when in relationship to meals etc. if you understand all this you are more likely to take it right.
(Woman, 49, diabetic, ibid.)

This opinion survey work is backed up by research evidence. In one study, 61 per cent of patients starting new medication reported unmet information needs after ten days (Barber *et al.*, 2004) . A National Audit Office study (Comptroller and Auditor General, 2003) provided evidence from doctors, pharmacists and patients that the information provided to patients on medicines is often confusing and inadequate . Research also demonstrates the positive difference that information can make: in a study of patients with chronic conditions in Europe and the USA, when patients receive health information on how to manage their condition, nearly two-thirds make proactive changes in behaviour based on the information. More than three-quarters of those who change their behaviour perceive a positive impact on their health (Pfizer, 2005).

It is important to remember that people have a broad range of preferences concerning information and that they want different information at different times (Raynor and Britten, 2001). As well as being highlighted in research, our own experience of developing information for patients has taught us that a 'one size fits all' approach does not work. Offering patients information in a way that they find helpful is about more than just explaining things more clearly. It is also a matter of asking about what they want to know and how they would like to receive it; for some people a printout of a high-quality page from the Internet may be ideal; others may prefer a web address; and yet others may want the telephone number of a patient organization support group or helpline that they can call. Information is most likely to be absorbed when patients perceive it to be relevant and tailored to them.

Practical experience has also highlighted the benefits of information that supports a dialogue between the health professional and patient over information given in isolation. It is just as important that patients feel confident about asking questions and engaging in a discussion as it is that they are able to access information about their condition and treatment. Many patients find it hard to be open with health professionals, and with doctors in particular there is still a perceived imbalance of power:

I sit in the car before I see my consultant and make a note of what I am going to say – and I have known her four or five years. I get so frightened that I won't be able to articulate what I want, especially as my condition is hormonal and I can't always control my emotions with the doctor. I have fought to be treated with respect. It's OK now. But I have had to fight to take my husband in with me. There seems no formal way for him to get reassurance. Also, it's an emotional thing and sometimes it's the person affected by my emotions that needs to explain.
(Woman, 40, Carter and Taylor, 2003)

There is a great awareness of the time pressures within the NHS, and many patients express concern about bothering health professionals unnecessarily or taking up too much time:

My doctor is very good but he just doesn't have time to tell you about these things [long-term effects of drugs]. He recommends them, but then he has a waiting room full of people.
(Levenson, 2002)

Some also have concerns that any difference of opinion or admission of problems will be viewed as undesirable behaviour. There is a fear of being stigmatized as difficult. In a project run by Age Concern (2004) , when patients were asked why they do not raise questions about their medicines with their doctor the most common responses given were:

'I don't want to be a nuisance.'
'I don't want to bother the doctor.'
'I would be challenging their professionalism.'
'They won't listen.'
'If I ask questions they might think I am being awkward.'

A discussion held during a focus group on medication review (Medicines Partnership, 2005) revealed that some patients are very worried indeed about what might happen if they told their doctor how they really feel:

Man: 'You should speak your mind. The doctor is a human being, same as you. Tell 'em how you feel inside.'
Woman: 'Yes, but it can go against you as anti-social behaviour.'
Man: 'That's right, they put it on your record as bad behaviour, and to me it's a free country and you should be able to speak your mind.'
Woman: 'I am very, very frightened.'

Several studies have supported this anecdotal evidence and shown that patients rarely fully voice their 'agendas' during consultations (Barry *et al.*, 2000) . The most commonly unvoiced issues are worries, ideas and information about their own lifestyle and social context. If patients fail to voice their doubts during the consultation, it can frequently lead to misunderstandings and miscommunication. Often patients will agree to take a prescription when they really plan to weigh up the pros and cons and make a decision about whether to follow it later on. This goes some way towards explaining why so many patients take away prescriptions that they then choose not to stick to.

To address this and make sure that patients are able to get the information they need from health professionals, it is important not only to improve the depth and quality of information about medicines, but also to change expectations so that asking questions about medicines becomes the norm. The concept of 'power questions' is one that is increasingly being explored in the UK to facilitate this change in culture (Medicines Partnership, 2005). It involves giving patients suggested questions, which they should feel comfortable about asking at any time. Examples of 'power questions' about medicines include:

- What does this medicine do?
- How long will I need to use it?
- How and when should I take it?
- Should I avoid any other medicines, drinks, foods or activities when I am taking this medicine?
- What are the possible risks and side-effects and what should I do if they happen to me?
- How do I know if this medicine is helping?
- What if I stopped taking it, or took a lower dose?
- Why do I need to carry on with this medicine if I am symptom-free?
- If I forget a dose, what should I do?
- Is there anything that can help remind me to take my medicines?

Displaying these questions in surgeries, pharmacies and hospitals or including them in patient information can be a great help in encouraging patients to be open about what they would like to talk about and in making sure that they have the right information to engage in an ongoing dialogue about their treatment.

These questions were developed for 'Ask About Medicines Week', a national campaign to improve communication between health professionals and patients about medicines. It is run by an independent organization and supported by an alliance of stakeholders including government, patient groups, health professionals, the pharmaceutical industry and the medicines regulator. It is funded from a mix of public and private sources.

'Ask About Medicines Week' demonstrates the value of a national multi-stakeholder campaign stimulating a wide range of local activities and developing new resources designed to enable people to access information about medicines and make better-informed choices about medicine-taking. More information about the initiative is available from www.askaboutmedicines.org.

Health professionals are prepared for partnership

There is a major culture change involved in empowering patients to engage as partners in decisions about treatment – a change that is already underway through the work of such initiatives as 'Ask About Medicines Week'. However, it is equally important that health professionals approach prescribing from a partnership perspective. This means viewing it as important to spend time listening to the patient's perspective and reaching an agreement, as well as having specific skills in communication and shared decision-making.

Patients say that, all too often, it feels as if health professionals are telling them what to do and are only interested in checking up on whether they are complying with instructions:

I think the meeting [medication review] with the pharmacist was to see, really, if you were mentally alert and taking your medication – the morning ones in the morning and the evening ones in the evening – being checked up on.
(Medicines Partnership, 2005)

It [medication review] was really to see if you needed help having your memory jogged to take this tablet or that tablet. That's the impression I got.
(Ibid.)

Research shows that, despite their best intentions, health professionals tend to be better at giving instructions than facilitating shared decisions (Makoul *et al.*, 1995). In one study that looked at discussions initiated by a doctor, 87 per cent of consultations involved doctors giving instructions for using a medication, but in only 15 per cent of cases did they ask the patient's opinion. Furthermore, the patient's ability to follow the treatment plan was only discussed in 5 per cent of cases. The strongest determinant of prescribing is the doctor's opinion about the patient's expectations of a prescription, and studies also show that GPs probably overestimate the patient's expectations of a prescription (Virji and Britten, 1991; Webb and Lloyd, 1994). Patients are up to ten times more likely to receive a prescription if the GP thinks that they expected one (Cockburn and Pitt, 1997). This means that exploring the patient's expectations and beliefs is key if unnecessary (in the opinion of the doctor) and unwanted (by the patient) prescriptions are to be avoided.

Experience in practice teaches that successful skills training must include the opportunity to try out techniques in a safe setting, preferably with patients involved and using a mix of real and simulated patients, video and role-play. And as well as developing communication skills, a key element is to develop an understanding of patients' perspectives. Communication skills are increasingly being developed as a core part of the syllabus for newly qualifying health professionals, and this trend should be encouraged and extended to encompass negotiation and shared decision-making.

Prescribing consultations involve patients as partners

Patients of all ages prefer to have some say in decisions about treatment and are currently not being involved as much as they want. A national survey (MORI, 2004) conducted in the UK asked people whether they generally prefer to make up their own mind about what treatment is right for them, to decide together with the doctor, or for the doctor to decide for them. In both 2003 and 2004, 24 per cent said that they would prefer to make up their own mind after the doctor had explained the options, 40 per cent would prefer to decide in partnership with the doctor, and 32 per cent would prefer the doctor to make the decision. In other words, *nearly two-thirds of patients want to be involved to some extent in decisions about their treatment.*

These proportions vary according to age, gender, geography and social class. In every category, at least half of the people prefer patient-centred decision-making to a traditional, paternalistic model where their doctor decides for them. For example, half of the over 65s, and 54 per cent of people from social classes D and E[1] want some say in decisions. More women than men want to be actively involved in choice of treatment, but 58 per cent of men still want to have some level of engagement. And whilst people in some parts of the North of England leant more strongly towards 'doctor knows best' than in the Midlands and the South, at least 53 per cent of patients in these areas wanted a partnership approach.

The goal is not to involve every patient in the decision about their medicine, but to make sure that everyone has the chance to be involved to the extent that they want. And there is still a long way to go: the 2004 Healthcare Commission patient survey in England found that 40 per cent of patients did not feel they were involved as much as they wanted to be in decisions about medicines and 30 per cent wanted to be more involved in decisions about care and treatment.

The stereotype of patients who want to take an active role in decisions may conjure up an image of young, well-educated, middle-class professionals from affluent areas. But it is a mistake to assume that older patients or people from less advantaged backgrounds do not want to have their say. More than anything, these data remind us that one size does not fit all.

This approach is increasingly being supported by evidence from research studies. There is no single clinical trial or set of trials that proves a definitive link between concordance in prescribing and improved health outcomes through better compliance. Rather, there is a growing and diverse evidence base that collectively supports the elements of concordance as being key to the effective use of medicines. This consists of evidence that single-factor interventions that do not involve patients in prescribing decisions (for example, providing additional written information alone) are unsuccessful (Peveler *et al.*, 1999), and emerging evidence that interventions that involve patients more are successful in improving both compliance and patient satisfaction (Dayan-Lintzer and Klein, 1999; Chambers *et al.*, 1999). This builds on numerous studies showing that patients' attitudes to risk and the extent to which they find side-effects tolerable can differ markedly from the assumptions made by health professionals, and that patients' beliefs and views about medicines are a key influence on whether and how they take them (LaRosa and LaRosa, 2000).

---

1. MORI defines social class D as working class (semi- and unskilled manual workers) and social class E as those at the lowest levels of subsistence (state pensioners and so on, with no other earnings).

Experience of supporting practical projects has shown that people value the opportunity to talk about their treatment with a health professional. Prompts and tools can help patients prepare for a consultation and talk about their concerns so that they feel able to come to a decision about what is best for them. Even an intervention as simple as encouraging a patient to write down the questions, concerns and issues which they would like to raise during a consultation, either with the pharmacist or with another health professional, can help.

Patient decision aids can be an effective way of helping patients become involved in decisions about their healthcare. They range from simple booklets to multi-media tools. What they have in common is the aim of helping patients prepare for a consultation with a health professional. They enable patients to make a better-informed choice based on personal values coupled with the clinical evidence, rather than promoting compliance with a single recommended option. The main objectives of decision aids are to enable patients to:

- understand the range of options available (both drug and other options)
- understand the probable consequences of options based on the best clinical evidence available
- consider the value they personally place on the consequences
- participate actively with healthcare professionals in deciding about options.

A recent Cochrane[2] review (O'Connor *et al*., 2003) concluded that trials show that decision aids improve knowledge and realistic expectations, enhance active participation in decision-making, lower decisional conflict, decrease the proportion of people remaining undecided, and improve agreement between values and choice.

Patients are supported in taking medicines

It is very important that patients have the opportunity to be fully prepared for, and engaged in, prescribing decisions. However, the prescribing consultation alone does not hold all the answers. It can be difficult to take in everything discussed at the consultation, and patients often need time to understand their condition and treatment:

> *More information on the medications [after a bypass] would be really useful, and there is a need for more education but the question is when. If you do too much beforehand it can frighten people. At the time of giving out the tablets the nurses are so busy. Also, at the time, I was in such a poor state that I wouldn't have taken it in.*
>
> (Man, 71, recovering from triple bypass, Carter and Taylor, 2003)

> *I was given all the information about the medication that I was going to be on, but you get the information at the wrong time, when you are very stressed. For example when you have been diagnosed with renal failure or when you are on dialysis. You get bombarded and it is difficult to retain the information. People may not remember that they have been told things.*
>
> (Man, 58, ibid.)

2. Cochrane reviews: These are written by the Cochrane Collaboration which is an international not-for-profit organization, providing up-to-date evidence-based information about the effects of healthcare.

It is important to look at what happens after a patient takes the medicine home, since issues often arise after a patient has been taking the medicine for a little while. Some patients find that when they feel better or get used to having a condition or taking a particular medicine they think of questions that had not initially occurred to them. For this reason, ongoing support plays a crucial role in helping patients to get the most out of their medicines, through delivering information at appropriate times, answering questions as they arise and providing practical support. Medication reviews provide one such opportunity and are welcomed by patients as an opportunity to ask questions: 'We'd like to ask all the things we couldn't ask when we were very ill' (Levenson, 2002).

Focus group work demonstrates that patients need preparation to get the most out of medication reviews. Many were not clear about the purpose of a review or about the potential benefits and had concerns that reviews were a cost-cutting measure or a covert compliance-monitoring exercise.

The past few years have seen the development of a number of patient support programmes which aim to help patients to get the most benefit from medicines after a prescribing decision has been made. Many of these programmes are funded by manufacturers, and these generally support a single drug. Others are provided on behalf of the health system as a whole, although up until now typically as research projects.

Patient support programmes come in many shapes and sizes, but the evidence suggests that the programmes most successful at improving compliance are those that provide a range of different support. In a Cochrane systematic review of the effectiveness of interventions to enhance compliance with all prescribed medicines 39 interventions were assessed (McDonald *et al.*, 2002). Of these, 19 showed significant increases in compliance and 17 showed significant improvements in outcome. The successful interventions shared characteristics – they were often complex and included combinations of enhanced conventional care, information, counselling, reminders, self-monitoring, reinforcement, family therapy and additional supervision or attention.

The Medicines Partnership is involved in piloting a number of patient support programmes. This experience echoes these findings: a single intervention is not enough, and ongoing support is needed. We have identified a number of features which characterize programmes that seem to be most effective in terms of helping patients to get the most benefit from treatment. Critically, such programmes must be interactive, work with patients' own views and beliefs and be flexible in meeting individual patients' information needs. Programmes work best where they listen and respond to patients' individual issues and concerns rather than push compliance messages, particularly where the programme only supports a single drug. For ethical reasons, patient enrolment in such programmes should also be voluntary.

Patient support programmes can be offered through a number of media – for example, inbound/outbound telephone calls, e-mail support, interactive websites, SMS text messages, newsletters and individual mailings. Telephone support, in particular, can be a cost-effective way of delivering an interactive service to address concerns on an ongoing basis and improve compliance. It has proved to be acceptable to patients (Car and Sheikh,

2003; Pinnock *et al.*, 2003; Kirman *et al.*, 1994; Johnston *et al.*, 2000; Maglavera *et al.*, 2002) and effective – for example, improving mood in depression (Hunkeler *et al.*, 2000). Such support has been used in asthma (MORI, 2004), diabetes (Schoen *et al.*, 2004), depression (Meresman *et al.*, 2003; Hunkeler *et al.*, 2000; Pearson *et al.*, 2003) and substance abuse (Parker *et al.*, 2002).

When delivered with these key principles in mind, support programmes can be very effective at meeting patients' information needs and increasing satisfaction:

> *The Helpline has been really useful and if I have any queries or concerns, I just ring them up and they will do everything they can to help me. The people on the other end of the phone are really nice, they understand what I feel like and I feel as if they really care, which sometimes I find a bit lacking in other areas. They also call me regularly to see how I am doing and if I have any problems, which is really reassuring.*[3]

Nurses and pharmacists are often very well placed to offer this sort of support and it can ease the burden on doctors' time and enhance the value of face-to-face follow-up appointments. Far from replacing the relationship that patients have with their health professionals, support programmes can help reinforce them. The most successful programmes encourage the patients to maintain a dialogue with their health professional so that action can be taken to deal with any issues identified as part of the programme. One patient on a telephone support programme commented:

> *I feel now that I understand my asthma treatments better which has come from both talking with you and going back to see my asthma nurse on your advice. She gave me permission to 'step-down' my inhaler treatment and also gave me some good leaflets.*[4]

CONCLUSION

At a time when more people are taking an ever-greater quantity of medicines, encouraging shared decision-making and helping patients to get the most out of their medicines is essential to avoid unnecessary ill-health as well as reduce waste and avoidable cost. What is clear from the research evidence and what patients tell us is that, in order to maximize the benefit of prescribed medicine, we need to move from the paternalistic model of 'doctor knows best' to a model in which patients are involved in decisions about treatment. Progress towards the effective use of medicines is only possible if key barriers to shared decision-making are overcome: it is not a quick fix and there is a need for a continuing culture shift towards involving patients, both in terms of patients being open about their beliefs and concerns and health professionals being committed to engaging patients as partners. In an environment of rising healthcare costs where non-compliance continues to be a problem, investing time in engaging patients in decisions and providing ongoing support is not just an option – it is a necessity.

3. Quote from a patient on the Biogen Avonex support programme. See http://www.medicines-partnership.org/projects/current-projects/avonex-support.
4. Quote from a patient on the Serum asthma support programme. See http://www.medicines-partnership.org/projects/current-projects/serum.

REFERENCES

Age Concern (2004), 'Can We Help You?' Project Report, Blackburn with Darwen, July, available at: http://www.medicines-partnership.org/medication-review/patient-feedback.

Barber, N., Parsons, J., Clifford, S., Darracott, R. and Horne, R. (2004), 'Patients' Problems with New Medication for Chronic Conditions', *Quality and Safety in Health Care*, **13**, pp. 172–75.

Barry, C.A., Bradley, C.P., Britten, N., Stevenson, F.A. and Barber, N. (2000), 'Patients' Unvoiced Agendas in General Practice Consultations: Qualitative Study', *British Medical Journal*, **320**, pp. 1246–50.

Car, J. and Sheikh, A. (2003), 'Telephone Consultations', *British Medical Journal*, **326**, pp. 966–99.

Carter, S. and Taylor, D. (2003), 'A Question of Choice: Compliance in Medicine Taking', Medicines Partnership, at: http://www.medicines-partnership.org/research-evidence/major-reviews/a-question-of-choice

Chambers, C.V., Markson, L., Diamond, J.J., Lasch, L. and Berger, M. (1999), 'Health Beliefs and Compliance with Inhaled Corticosteroids by Asthmatic Patients in Primary Care Practices', *Respiratory Medicine*, **93**(2), pp. 88–94.

Cockburn, J. and Pitt, S. (1997), 'Prescribing Behaviour in Clinical Practice: Patients' Expectations and Doctors' Perceptions of Patients' Expectations – A Questionnaire Study', *British Medical Journal*, **315**, pp. 520–23.

Comptroller and Auditor General (2003), *Safety, Quality and Efficacy: Regulating Medicines in the UK*, January, London: National Audit Office, available at: http://www.nao.org.uk/publications/nao_reports/02-03/0203255.pdf (accessed June 2006).

Dayan-Lintzer, M. and Klein, P. (1999), 'Galenic, Concerted Choice and Compliance with HRT', *Contraception, Fertilité, Sexualité*, **27**(4), pp. 318–21.

Department of Health (2001), *National Service Framework for Older People*, available at: http://www.dh.gov.uk/PublicationsAndStatistics/fs/en

Department of Health (2003), *Prescriptions Dispensed in the Community. Statistics for 1993–2003*: England, available at: http://www.dh.gov.uk/PublicationsAndStatistics/fs/en.

Department of Health (2005), *Better Information, Better Choices, Better Health*, available at: http://www.dh.gov.uk.

Dillner, L. (1996), 'Pill Scare Linked to Rise in Abortions', *British Medical Journal*, **312**(996), 20 April, available at: http://www.bmj.com.

Farmer, R.D., Williams, T.J., Simpson, E.L. and Nightingale, A.L. (2000), 'Effect of 1995 Pill Scare on Rates of Venous Thromboembolism among Women Taking Combined Oral Contraceptives: Analysis of General Practice Research Database', *British Medical Journal*, **321**(7259), 19–26 August, pp. 477–79.

Healthcare Commission (2004), *Primary Care Trust Survey 2004 (England)*, available at: http://www.healthcarecommission.org.uk/nationalfindings/surveys/patientsurveys/nationalnhssurveyprogramme2004.

Horne, R. and Weinman, J. (1999), 'Patients' Beliefs about Prescribed Medicines and their Role in Adherence to Treatment in Chronic Illness', *Journal of Psychosomatic Research*, **47**(6), pp. 555–67.

Hunkeler, E. *et al.* (2000), 'Efficacy of Nurse Telehealth Care and Peer Support in Augmenting Treatment of Depression in Primary Care', *Archives of Family Medicine*, **9**, pp. 700–708.

Johnston, B. *et al.* (2000), 'Outcomes of the Kaiser Permanente Tele–Home Health Research Project', *Archives of Family Medicine*, **9**, pp. 40–45.

Kirman, M. *et al.* (1994), 'A Telephone-delivered Intervention for Patients with NIDDM – Effect on Coronary Risk Factors', *Diabetes Care*, **17**, pp. 840–46.

LaRosa, J.H. and LaRosa, J.C. (2000), 'Enhancing Drug Compliance in Lipid-lowering Treatment, *Archives of Family Medicine*, **9**, pp. 1169–75.

Levenson, R. (2002), *Medication Reviews – The Views of Patients*, a report to the Medicines Partnership, available at: http://www.medicines-partnership.org/medication-review/room-for-review/downloads.

McDonald, H., Garg, A. and Haynes, R. (2002), 'Interventions to Enhance Patient Adherence to Medication Prescriptions', *Journal of the American Medical Association*, **288**, pp. 2868–79.

Maglavera, N. *et al.* (2002), 'Home Care Delivery through the Mobile Telecommunications Platform', *International Journal of Medical Informatics*, **68**, pp. 99–111.

Makoul, G., Arntson, P. and Schofield, T. (1995), 'Health Promotion in Primary Care: Physician–Patient Communication and Decision Making about Prescription Medications', *Social Science and Medicine*, **41**(9), pp. 1241–54.

Medicines Partnership (2005), *Implementing Medication Review: An Evaluation of the Impact of 'Room for Review'*, available at: http://www.medicines-partnership.org/medication-review/room-for-review/impact-evaluation.

Meresman, J. *et al.* (2003), 'Implementing a Nurse Telecare Program for Treating Depression in Primary Care', *Psychiatry Quarterly*, **74**, pp. 61–73.

MORI (2004), *The Public and Prescribed Medicines 2004*, research sponsored by the Medicines Partnership, available at: http://www.medicines-partnership.org.

O'Connor, A.M., Stacey, D., Entwistle, V., Llewellyn-Thomas, H. *et al.* (2003), 'Decision Aids for People Facing Health Treatment or Screening Decisions (Cochrane Review)', in *The Cochrane Library*, Issue 3, Update Software, Oxford.

Parker, J., Turk, C. and Busby, L. (2002), 'A Brief Telephone Intervention Targeting Treatment Engagement from a Substance Abuse Program Wait List', *Journal of Behaviour and Health Services Research*, **29**, pp. 288–303.

Pearson, B. *et al.* (2003), 'Evidence-based Care for Depression in Maine: Dissemination of the Kaiser Permanente Nurse Telecare Program', *Psychiatry Quarterly*, **74**, pp. 91–102.

Peveler, R., George, C., Kinmouth, A.L., Campbell, M. and Thomson, C. (1999), 'Effect of Antidepressant Drug Counselling and Information Leaflets on Adherence to Drug Treatment in Primary Care: Randomised Controlled Trial', *British Medical Journal*, **319**, pp. 612–15.

Pfizer (2005), *The Informed Patient. Quantitative Research among Patients in Europe and the USA* (further details unavailable).

Pinnock, H. *et al.* (2003), 'Accessibility, Acceptability and Effectiveness in Primary Care of Routine Telephone Review of Asthma: Pragmatic, Randomised Controlled Trial', *British Medical Journal*, **326**, pp. 477–81.

Raynor, D.K. and Britten, N. (2001), 'Medicines Information Leaflets Fail Concordance Test, *British Medical Journal*, **322**, p. 1541.

Schoen, C., Osborn, R., Huynh, P.T., Doty, M., Davis, K., Zapert, K. and Peugh, J. (2004), 'Primary Care and Health System Performance: Adults' Experiences in Five Countries', *Health Affairs*, 28 October, available at: http://content.healthaffairs.org/cgi/content/abstract/hlthaff.w4.487 (accessed June 2006).

Virji, A. and Britten, N. (1991), 'A Study of the Relationship between Patients' Attitudes and Doctors Prescribing', *Family Practice*, **8**, pp. 314–19.

Webb, S. and Lloyd, M. (1994), 'Prescribing and Referral in General Practice: A Study of Patients' Expectations and Doctors' Actions', *British Journal of General Practice*, 44, pp. 165–69.

CHAPTER 13

The Role of the Expert Patient in Compliance and Concordance

Brendan O'Rourke

The aims of this chapter are:

- To outline the concept of lay-led self-management for people living with long-term conditions.
- To contextualize the concept historically.
- To locate self-management within a social model of health.
- To examine strategies used on self-management courses that may impact on the issue of compliance.
- To demonstrate that courses are vehicles to develop self-efficacy, improved confidence levels and feelings of control.
- To describe emerging trends which seem to indicate improved levels of confidence and lead to better communication between healthcare professionals and people with long-term conditions.
- To outline the steps necessary for the development of successful lay-led self-management programmes.

A set of thoughts often voiced to UK primary care trust (PCT) [1] gatherings these days goes as follows:

1. Since April 2002, PCTs have taken control of local healthcare in the UK while 28 new strategic health authorities monitor performance and standards. The 302 PCTs, covering all parts of England, receive budgets directly from the Department of Health.

What would you say if there arrived in the National Health Service (NHS) a treatment which had been demonstrated, in randomized controlled trials, to have significant beneficial effect when administered to people living with a range of long-term health conditions?
Factor in that the treatment has been useful in helping symptoms from physical conditions and mild depression or 'the blues' arising from having a condition. It is usually administered on a generic basis to groups of people with varied long-term conditions, with significant improvements shown in symptom relief and in people's confidence to manage their daily lives.
Would you be interested?

Now factor in that the treatment is administered in one discrete course lasting six weeks – with no negative side-effects. It has been shown to have beneficial effects lasting up to three years after the initial course. And as an interesting side-effect, health professionals frequently find that they enjoy a more constructive relationship with people who have undertaken the course. People who have experienced the treatment seem to develop a more positive attitude to life and a willingness to take an active part in managing their health.

This is not a drug – if it were, pharmaceutical companies would be bottling it and selling it at premium prices. This is EPP – the Expert Patients Programme.

The EPP hit the ground running when it arrived in the NHS. The first cohort of staff recruited in 2002 was based across England – approximately one team of two people to each strategic health authority (SHA) area. Most were new to the NHS and many were from the voluntary sector. Some primary care trusts agreed to house the new staff in offices they could identify from their stock. Other staff worked without an office for over a year. Despite backing from key stakeholders within the NHS and Department of Health, notably the Chief Medical Officer (CMO), there was no grand publicity or marketing campaign to accompany the launch. Staff had to design their own leaflets, recruit volunteers to train the course from diverse sources in communities, and train them to deliver the Programme. At the same time, a whole new approach and philosophy was being introduced in the NHS – to the advantage of health professionals and managers but, above all, to people living with long-term conditions.

Assets the Programme had were backing from the Department of Health and a training and quality team with experience of driving successful programmes in the voluntary sector.

Three years down the line about 30 000 people with long-term conditions have been through EPPs, and over 1000 volunteer course tutors have been recruited and trained to deliver the module to a standard consistent with the quality framework.

The self-management approach is based on a social model of health that places people who are living with long-term conditions centre-stage as decision-makers in the management of their health. This is not surprising, really – all the EPP staff recruited are themselves living with long-term conditions, or have experience, gained from an informal caring role, of behaviour change which has allowed patients to become the decision-makers.

WHY BOTHER TO INVOLVE PATIENTS? DON'T WE JUST WANT COMPLIANCE?

The question may be phrased, why bother worrying? If it's not broken, don't fix it – why not make do with the modernist-type twentieth-century approach, viewing all patients as passive recipients of care and not as decision-makers? Have not physicians always sought to ensure that patients understand the importance of complying with their treatment plan? It is useful to take a view of the wider social and demographic climate in which the NHS has operated. In its early years and at the height of the purported 'Butskellite' consensus in social policy – named after the Labour leader Hugh Gaitskell and Conservative Minister Rab Butler – the NHS was focused more on addressing acute, rather than long-term, conditions. Access to good medical treatment free at the point of delivery was, for most people, a fairly recent innovation. The NHS was, as it still remains, hugely popular among people with a not-too-distant folk memory of privation in sickness. A typical model for the role of a patient with an acute condition was often seen to be that of deference to medical judgement and dutiful compliance with a given treatment regime, in the hope of a 'cure' and a return to civil society.

Much has changed: patterns of deference have declined, and a more questioning attitude is taken towards the institutions of governance and the welfare state. Medical professionals have voiced concern that issues of clinical discretion for the best interests of the patient in prescribing decisions have to be balanced against managerial issues of resource constraint.

There is increased consumerism of choice in healthcare:

> *Patients are increasingly involved in making decisions about their health care (for example, using interactive video discs for medical decision making and home monitoring devices to measure blood pressure). As patients become better informed, change in the traditional doctor-patient relationship is inevitable.*
>
> (Towle, 1998, p. 302)

Demographic change has brought about an attendant switch in prevalent disease pattern. More of the work of the NHS is now taken up by the management of long-term conditions. Symptoms may develop over time, diagnosis is tentative and there is often no single cure, nor indeed one single model of treating the condition. The job of the prescribing physician is less a matter of administering a treatment which will lead to a cure, and more often one of agreeing with an informed patient the treatment plans and strategies which will lead to an optimized quality of life.

A new challenge is to recognize the expertise of both parties in the consulting room – that is, the expertise of the physician in application of medical technique, and that of the person with a long-term condition in living with the condition and developing coping strategies. Unless the expertise of both is recognized and a more equal balance of power achieved, problem issues may not be limited to communication.

The problematic nature of compliance has been widely documented, ranging from the extent of non-compliance across disease types to a critical examination of the definition itself. Dunbar and Jacob (2001) stated that up to 80 per cent of patients may be non-compliant with treatment regime, although the extent differs across disease type (quoted in Carter and Taylor, 2003, p. 9). Other sources note the importance of psychosocial issues and belief about medicine-taking in influencing compliance.

Carter and Taylor (2003, p. 11) state: 'There is a strong case for concluding that compliance-related interventions should be designed to help the patient make an informed choice about their medicine taking, rather than "improve compliance" per se'.

WHAT DO WE WANT?

The 1999 White Paper, *Saving Lives: Our Healthier Nation*, noted the success of the voluntary organization Arthritis Care in developing 'Challenging Arthritis', a self-management programme for condition-specific groups (Department of Health, 1999, para. 3.44). People who had been through the programme, introduced to the country by Jean Thompson and her colleagues, were not only able to use their experience to help others as well as themselves, but were also able to take more control of their lives and make best use of professional advice. Jean Thompson was to become one of the principal trainers of the Expert Patients Programme, alongside Jim Phillips. The 1999 White Paper committed the government to develop a patient-led self-management programme:

> *People with chronic illnesses are often in the best position to know how to cope. There is increasing evidence from research studies and from patients' associations that people have improved health and reduced incapacity if they take the lead themselves in managing their chronic disease – with good support from the health service.*
> (Department of Health, 1999, para. 3.49)

One of the twelve ways in which people were found to be able to help themselves after participation in a self-management programme was in correctly using medication (derived from Lorig *et al.*, 1999). However, the main benefits were increased feelings of confidence and control, plus the ability to plan ahead and a more constructive relationship with health professionals.

An Expert Patients Programme was heralded in the NHS Plan of July 2000, and a task force set up with Professor Liam Donaldson as chair. *The Expert Patient: A New Approach to Chronic Disease Management for the 21st Century* was released by the Department of Health in 2001. The report noted the aforesaid demographic shift that had taken place in the latter part of the twentieth century, and that, with more people living into their 70s and 80s, the predominant pattern of disease had changed. Most of the time and budget of the NHS was now being taken up with the management of long-term conditions, such as heart disease, diabetes mellitus, chronic obstructive pulmonary disease, cancer and mental illness. For many long-term conditions there was still no cure.

The report noted: 'In Great Britain, at any one time, as many as 17.5 million adults may be living with a chronic disease. Older people suffer more with up to three quarters of people aged 75 and older falling into this category' (Department of Health, 2001, p. 4). It called for a change of emphasis, noting that, even in the better services, the impetus had been on provision of information, giving advice and answering questions. Few had moved beyond this to a model where self-management of a long-term condition was considered a valid option. In this respect, the report called for a fundamental shift:

> *... [to] encourage and enable patients to take an active role in their own care... Patient self-management programmes, or Expert Patient Programmes, are not simply about educating or instructing patients about their condition and then measuring success on the basis of patient compliance. They are based on developing the confidence and motivation of patients to use their own skills and knowledge to take effective control over life with a chronic illness.*
>
> (Ibid., p.5)

The report went on to talk about the commonalities of experience among many people living with diverse long-term conditions:

> *People have problems specific to their individual illness but there is also a core of common needs: for example knowing how to recognise and act upon symptoms, dealing with acute attacks or exacerbations of the disease, making the most effective use of medicines and treatments, dealing with fatigue, managing work and developing strategies to deal with the psychological consequences of the disease.*
>
> (Ibid., p. 4)

The task force recommended establishing a national network of lay-led self-management trainers under the auspices of the NHS in England. The first trainers were appointed the following year. But in the decade preceding the report, a great deal of good practice had already been developed.

WHERE DOES LAY-LED SELF-MANAGEMENT COME FROM?

> *It was the best thing that happened to me for many years. It allowed me to express all the things that I had bottled up for a long time. It allowed me to talk, listen and learn and gave me 'survival' techniques for this illness.*
>
> (Quote from a participant on a self-management course, Long-Term Medical Conditions Alliance)

Self-management involves dealing with the consequence of the illness from the standpoint of the person with the condition. The approach complements good medical care and does not attempt to be a substitute. It is about problem-solving, confidence-building, decision-making and improving communication between patients and medical professionals to form a real partnership. Although it was new to the NHS in 2001, there was already a wealth of experience and research evidence in the voluntary sector.

The organization Arthritis Care was a pioneer in the field in 1994. Under the programme

'Challenging Arthritis' it trained groups of people with arthritis in a course developed at Stanford University in the USA.

Professor Kate Lorig developed the first arthritis-based training programmes at Stanford. She found that groups of people with arthritis could be motivated to change their behaviours by participating in training modules where information was given in bite-sized chunks. Trained volunteers living with the condition could deliver the programmes.

The self-management approach was developed further in the voluntary sector, and government funding was supplied for the Long-Term Medical Conditions Alliance (LMCA) to coordinate a 'Living Well' project. This project used as its core module the generic Chronic Disease Self-Management Course. The CDSMC had been developed by Kate Lorig at Stanford after the arthritis-specific course. The commonality of experience of people with long-term conditions was being appreciated; many people with arthritis trained on the original course were found to have co-morbidities, and the course deals with symptoms as opposed to the disease. Medical questions raised by attendees on courses are referred back to the medical professionals on all Stanford-based self-management courses: the Chronic Disease Self-Management Course, Arthritis Self-Management Course and Positive Self-Management Course (for people affected by HIV).

The research base on benefits looked at by the Expert Patient task force was impressive. There had been over 100 studies across three continents. Typical outcomes in the USA have included reduced severity of symptoms, improvement in self-efficacy and psychological state, increased use of health-promoting techniques, improved communication with doctors and reduction in visits to doctors or to accident and emergency departments (emergency rooms). Overall the US research showed that a 5 per cent increase in self-care led to a 20 per cent decrease in professional care (Kemper *et al.*, 1993).

Professor Julie Barlow from the Psychosocial Research Centre at Coventry University reviewed all the research for the Expert Patient report. In her own research for the LMCA project, the comparison of outcomes at four months compared to baseline showed significant increases on cognitive symptom management, disease self-efficacy, communication with doctors and general rating of mental health. Significant decreases were found on fatigue, health distress and visits to specialists over the four-month period (Barlow *et al.* in Cooper, 2001). As one patient on the project commented, 'It gave me a more positive feeling about myself, better self-esteem' (ibid., p. 44).

The CDSMC is the core module being used in the roll-out phase of the EPP, which trainers are delivering in the community and training volunteer course tutors to deliver. It is a generic, as opposed to disease-specific, module, although there have been some disease-specific pilots – for instance, for aphasia, mental illness and learning difficulties.

The course runs for two and a half hours per session for six weekly sessions. Sessions act as building-blocks to self-efficacy. It takes place in a community, rather than medical, venue and is delivered by two tutors who have been trained to deliver the course and who themselves have long-term conditions. No prior medical knowledge or expertise is expected of tutors before they are trained, beyond experience of behaviour change through living with a long-term condition. Tutors with different long-term conditions may train participants with a variety of other conditions – the focus is on addressing problems, not dealing with the specifics of the condition. Most groups range in size from 12 to 16 participants.

The tutors follow a tightly scripted manual to ensure quality. The generic course focuses on the shared experiences of people with a range of conditions, and problem areas from the individual's standpoint such as pain, fatigue, depression, fear of the future, and poor communication with medical professionals.

The generic course aims to provide people with a toolkit of skills to encourage health-promoting behaviours, build confidence and increase self-efficacy. The course content deals with goal-setting and action-planning, exercise, symptom management techniques, communication and proper use of medication. The process by which it is taught is as important as the content.

WHY DOES IT WORK?

Some elements of the training may seem to bear direct relevance to compliance. Carter and Taylor (2003, p. 7) have summarized a number of key points affecting compliance. They state that 'medicines taken for preventive purposes are especially likely not to be taken as prescribed'. Other factors were unwanted side-effects, concern about the value or appropriateness of taking medicines in particular contexts, complex medicine regimes and confusion.

On one level, that of information-giving, reliable health information is given in a controlled environment in which participants learn cognitive symptom management techniques. Communication skills are covered on week four, and then participants are invited to outline a problem that they are currently having with communication in a problem-solving session. It is significant that the literature on compliance notes that this is a difficult area of study because health service users 'often find it difficult to be honest with health care professionals about how they really take medicines' (Carter and Taylor, 2003, p. 85).

Medication usage is covered on week five of the CDSMC. Participants are taken through the purposes of medication, and then the negative effects of some medications are outlined: no apparent effect, allergy, side-effects and antagonistic effects of several medications in the event of co-morbidities. The responsibilities of taking medication are outlined, as is the importance of good communication with health professionals in the event of non-compliance. Course participants generate ideas for remembering to take medications that have been prescribed.[2]

2. Stanford Patient Education Research Centre: Kate Lorig, RN; Dr P.H. Virginia González, MPH; Diana Laurent, MPH; *Chronic Disease Self-Management Course Tutors Manual, 1997* – as adapted by Jim Phillips and Jean Thompson.

On the same week participants are given a toolkit for making informed treatment decisions for any treatment – mainstream medical as well as complementary or alternative treatments. The following week, on the sixth and final week of the course, there is an activity on informing the healthcare team, reporting health trends and developing constructive relationships with healthcare professionals.

But that is not the bigger picture, because provision of information can only go so far. The main focus of the course is to develop self-efficacy; giving people the confidence, as well as the knowledge and skills, to set achievable goals and use the information that is available.

Knowing something is only the first step. The key is moving people to action. To illustrate: there are things we all 'know' will be good for us as individuals or as a community, from recycling all rubbish to taking adequate exercise, from eating lots of fresh fruit and vegetables to putting enough by for our pensions. Knowledge does not necessarily lead to behaviour change. To build confidence in people's ability to change to more health-promoting behaviours, at each session course participants are invited to share with the group an action plan for the week ahead that should be feasible, behaviour-specific, planned in their schedule and, above all, something they want to do themselves. The plan should not be something that a participant thinks the doctor, or their family or the trainers want them to do, but something they themselves want to do.

The trainers model completion of feasible action plans and, with the group, practise other self-efficacy-enhancing techniques, such as persuasion and positive reinforcement when plans have been achieved.

If plans have been unsuccessful, or too ambitious, the group takes part in a problem-solving session to deal with the underlying issue. The trainers do not allow evaluation or cutting down of the different ideas generated to solve the problem, but ask the person concerned if any of the ideas has been helpful.

The prime importance of self-efficacy in achieving goals was developed from the work of Albert Bandura at Stanford University on social learning theory (Bandura, 1997). Social learning theory (or social cognitive theory) has stressed the importance of modelling and observational learning: 'What people think, believe, and feel affects how they behave. The natural and extrinsic effects of their actions, in turn, partly determine their thought patterns and affective reactions' (Bandura, 1985, p. 25). Bandura goes on to state:

> *People's conceptions about themselves and the nature of things are developed and verified through four different processes: direct experience of the effects produced by their actions, vicarious experience of the effects produced by somebody else's actions, judgments voiced by others, and derivation of further knowledge from what they already know by using rules of inference.*
>
> (Ibid., p. 27)

When a participant on the course works with the trainers to set an achievable action plan, and receives positive reinforcement from the group for their success, confidence levels are raised. If a member of the group is unsuccessful they receive motivation from the group to modify the plan and celebrate success.

By the end of the six-week course most group members have raised confidence levels and feel that they have gained new skills in cognitive symptom management. Typically, they will feel more prepared for medical consultations and are able to participate and communicate their needs on a more equal basis.

The interim monitoring results for EPPs in England find that 94 per cent of people feel that attending the course was a positive experience. Comments from a course participant from East Kent Coastal illustrate the importance of motivational action planning:

These meetings have provided a very positive experience for me. This has been due to the professional approach of all who have been involved in facilitating the course. Ongoing encouragement, sensitivity and understanding have been present at each point of contact, both at PCT and Tutor level, and at the learning Centre. The course structure has been well balanced and comprehensive, and the group process expertly managed. I have moved from an initial position of very low self-esteem, that of being a 'shadow of my former self', to a progressive gaining of confidence. Most importantly, at this time, I have increased hope for the future. I now have a strong sense of achievement and an increased desire to continue to move forwards. The weekly Action Plan has provided a basis for me to implement change. This element has given me the motivation to bring forward and reintroduce good practice for living, and to complement previous learning. The accompanying handbook has provided clearly presented reference material throughout. The opportunities for me to listen to, and share with, other course participants have been much appreciated. Running within the regular and well-defined framework of tutor input, these have enabled me to share relevant experiences with others. I have also been able to continue working on raising my level of self-awareness, control and effectiveness.
(Participant on the East Kent Coastal PCT)

A participant from Dartford, Gravesend and Swanley makes similar points, but also addresses the effect of having a long-term condition on social and emotional factors:

I have attended all 6 sessions of the course (which of the first 2, I wasn't sure that it was for me). I still carried on going and glad that I did. As I feel that this course has really helped me. The main thing I feel that it does is certainly open your eyes. I learnt by planning my time and achieving things, rather than putting things off or saying I can't do that. Also I tended to forget about how the family were feeling. So doing an action plan really helped to sort the problems out. I actually felt a lot better in myself knowing that I had achieved most of the things that I had set out to do. My family have also benefited by this course and tell me that I have changed by doing it. If that was all I got out of it then it really was worth doing. I have found by doing the course also that for me the relaxation part really works. I would never have done this and now do it several times a week and benefit so much from it. I do feel the course has been beneficial and hope others feel the same.
(Course participant from Dartford, Gravesend and Swanley)

So the prime driver of self-management is to develop self-efficacy, by prioritizing the experience of people with a long-term condition and validating their knowledge as experts at living with the condition. What steps need to be made to implement a self-management programme and how has it fared in the NHS?

HOW TO INSTITUTE A SELF-MANAGEMENT PROGRAMME

The EPP works from a social model of health and, as such, is rare in the NHS where a medical model prevails. EPP teams consisting of two trainers were appointed within each SHA area during the pilot period from 2002 to 2004/5. Their job was to train courses and to recruit two volunteer tutors for training per PCT area. PCTs received the cost of training two volunteers and £1200 to stage the first four courses. The trainers were also tasked with ensuring cross-boundary working, liaison with the voluntary sector and supporting new approaches.

In the transitional period, 2005–2008, there is a shift of emphasis. The task now is to develop each PCT's capacity to deliver courses in its area, and support the mainstreaming agenda while retaining responsibility for the Stanford Licence, under which the CDSMC is delivered, and quality requirements.

The success of EPPs has contributed to self-management being featured in successive recent documents and policy announcements. *Supporting People with Long Term Conditions, An NHS and Social Care Model to Support Local Innovation and Integration*, released by the Department of Health on 5 January 2005, states:

> *The Expert Patient Programme (EPP) has been central in spreading good self care and self management skills to a wider range of people with long term conditions. The programme provides group-based, generic training and is delivered by a network of trainers and volunteer tutors all living with long term conditions themselves. The EPP will be made available through all PCTs by 2008.*
>
> *By increasing the amount of information available to patients, health and social care providers can empower them to take better care of themselves and their own conditions. The EPP pilots and other local initiatives to support self care and self management have highlighted the need to pro-actively engage patients. This is not only about getting the right patients involved. It is also about ensuring that once they are 'through the door' they receive relevant and accessible information that meets their diverse needs.*
>
> (Department of Health, 2005, p. 31)

The *NHS Improvement Plan* of June 2004 also stated that EPP will be rolled out throughout the NHS by 2008 'enabling thousands more patients to take control of their own health and their own lives' (Department of Health, 2004, p. 40).

A research team from Manchester, York and Bristol Universities, comprising the National Primary Care Research and Development Centres, is conducting a randomized controlled trial of up to 1000 people from around the country and from different geographic and demographic groups who have been through courses.. The research will be available from 2006. However, the Department of Health has released indicative data from its own internal monitoring, which may reveal emergent trends. This research was summarized by Jane Cooper, EPP Projects Manager for Partnerships and Quality in the document *Stepping Stones to Success: An Implementation, Training and Support Framework for Lay Led Self Management Programmes* (Cooper, 2005).

EPP Pilot internal evaluation
Data from approximately 1000 EPP participants who completed the course between January 2003 and January 2005 indicate that the programme is achieving its aims.

Providing significant numbers of people with long-term conditions with the confidence and skills to better manage their condition on a daily basis.

- 45% said that they felt more confident that common symptoms (pain, tiredness, depression and breathlessness) would no longer interfere with their lives.
- 38% felt that such symptoms were less severe four to six months after completing the course.
- 33% felt better prepared for consultations with health professionals.

Providing significant reductions in service usage by people with long-term conditions completing the EPP course.

- 7% reductions in GP consultations.
- 10% reductions in outpatient visits.
- 16% reductions in Accident & Emergency Attendances.
- 9% reductions in Physiotherapy use. (Cooper, 2005, p. 5)

Increased confidence levels in symptom management, combined with people feeling better prepared for meeting health professionals, are therefore significant emerging trends.

This document goes on to set out the four key stepping stones to successful implementation of a self-management programme, in the NHS or in voluntary organizations. There are consistent standards of accreditation and quality across sectors. The first stepping stone stresses adherence to the values and principles of lay-led self-management – a core value being that 'the people who know most about the day-to-day problems of living with a long term condition are people living with long term conditions' (Cooper, 2005, p. 8). Programmes should be empowering vehicles for self-efficacy, and the integrity of the process should not be lost in implementation.

Programmes cannot be said to be empowering within communities if they serve to replicate and reinforce existing patterns of social and health inequality. The EPP has a diverse workforce and has made significant efforts to reach a representative spread of participants. The very first cohort of participants on courses saw a relative overrepresentation of people who were confident enough to engage in group activities, and these tended to be white, female and middle-class. This had also been an issue in the voluntary sector – perhaps inevitably, as early adopters are often people who are already keyed into networks. The *Stepping Stones* document has as a core value that 'Programmes should be delivered at grass roots level, in the first instance, by volunteer tutors recruited across all groups in the community' and that 'Efforts should be made to gain representation from all voices within communities' (Cooper, 2005, p. 9). This will be crucial as the Programme moves from pilot to mainstreaming.

Birmingham PCTs are working with the SHA to address issues of health inequality by giving added weighting to participants from wards with high levels of social deprivation. Specialist courses are being developed for people with aphasia and mental illness, and the course has been translated into a number of community languages, including Urdu, Hindi, Turkish, Punjabi and Greek for delivery by bilingual trainers. The EPP is working with the voluntary sector and with minority ethnic community organizations, such as Social Action for Health in Tower Hamlets, who first translated the course for the Bengali community.

Other stepping stones for the success of a self-management programme are to generate support in the organization and community, and appoint a self-management coordinator to be a champion, organize networks and courses and be a point of contact for the volunteers. Self-management is a cost-effective and inexpensive intervention, but it cannot be done for free. Successful programmes are those which have received the investment required and been given the right level of managerial expertise.

The fourth and final stepping stone to success is to recruit, train and support people living with long-term conditions to deliver courses. Tutors should be recruited from a range of cultural backgrounds to act as role models for self-efficacy, and representation sought from all voices within communities.

Of course, the course is not a panacea for all ills and will not be a suitable intervention for everyone. For example, this is not an intervention best suited to people who are newly diagnosed with a condition, as they may not be ready to deal with the fact that they have a condition they have to manage long-term. A self-management course, trained through the EPP or the voluntary sector, may be appropriate if they find it difficult later on to adhere to their agreed treatment plan.

Also, not everyone can commit to attend six weekly two-and- a-half-hour sessions, or be willing to attend group interventions. The roll-out of the EPP Online Pilot Project, an Internet-based version of the course, is designed to assist people who don't wish to attend a course in the community to access self-management skills.

Self-referral is a key aspect of the approach – people have to *want* to self-manage. Communities are being made aware of the approach from a wide range of sources, from articles in newspapers and health magazines to radio features, leaflets and community launches. The national EPP network is in place until the end of the pilot, and each PCT should have an EPP lead.

The national picture in PCTs is as yet uneven. More work needs to be done to integrate the social model of health with the medical and biopsychosocial models. An approach which places the person with a long-term condition at the centre of the system is preferable to a maze of unidisciplinary care pathways focused around the needs of services. However, the government is committed to rolling out the EPP throughout the NHS so that, by 2008, thousands more people will have been able to access the benefits of self-management within a mainstreamed service.

CONCLUSIONS

Demographic factors and wider sociocultural change have necessitated a change in the traditional relationship between healthcare professionals and people seeking their services:

- A primary driver of change has been in patterns of disease over the latter years of the last century. Most of the work of the NHS became focused on the needs of people with long-term, as opposed to acute, conditions.
- User-led self-management as a healthcare intervention of benefit to people with long-term conditions has built up a sound evidence base overseas and in the UK in the voluntary sector.
- Self-management works from a social model of health, and the integrity of the process is crucial to its success.
- People attending self-management courses receive reliable information on medication usage, treatment decisions and strategies to improve communication with healthcare professionals.
- The main benefit of self-management is in developing feelings of self-efficacy – peoples' beliefs about their own strengths and abilities to take control over their lives, set and achieve feasible goals, solve problems and deal with the challenges they face.
- Self-management courses are delivered by lay volunteers who themselves have long-term conditions, to groups of up to 16 people in non-medical settings. The volunteers model self-management of their condition to the group and use other self-efficacy-enhancing techniques.
- Emerging trends indicate that people attending user-led self-management courses develop feelings of confidence and strategies to cope with symptoms, and improve communication with healthcare professionals in a more constructive and equal relationship.
- The NHS and organizations licensed to deliver Stanford-based self-management courses should adhere to the agreed ways of working, principles and good practice that have developed over the years in the voluntary sector and in the EPP in order to sustain the benefits of the approach as it is mainstreamed.

REFERENCES

Bandura, A. (1985), *Social Foundations of Thought and Action: A Social-Cognitive Theory*, New York: Prentice Hall.

Bandura, A. (1997), *Self-Efficacy: The Exercise of Control*, New York: W.H. Freeman.

Carter, S. and Taylor, D. (2003), 'A Question of Choice: Compliance in Medicine Taking, Medicines Partnership', at: http://www.medicines-partnership.org/research-evidence/major-reviews/a-question-of-choice.

Cooper, J. (2001), *Partnerships for Successful Self Management: The Report of the Living with Long Term Illness Project*, London: LMCA.

Cooper J. (2005), *Stepping Stones to Success: An Implementation, Training and Support Framework for Lay Led Self Management Programmes*, Department of Health, London: Stationery Office.

Department of Health (1999), *Saving Lives: Our Healthier Nation*, London: Stationery Office.

Department of Health (2001), *The Expert Patient: A New Approach to Chronic Disease Management for the 21st Century*, London: Stationery Office.

Department of Health (2004), *The NHS Improvement Plan*, London: Stationery Office.

Department of Health (2005), *Supporting People with Long Term Conditions: An NHS and Social Care Model to Support Local Innovation and Integration*, London: Stationery Office.

Kemper, D.W., Lorig, K.L. and Mettler, M. (1993), 'The Effectiveness of Medical Self Care Interventions: A Focus on Self-initiated Responses to Symptoms', *Patient Education and Counseling*, **21**, pp. 29–39.

Lorig, K.L. *et al.* (1999), 'Evidence Suggesting that a Chronic Disease Self-Management Program Can Improve Health Status While Reducing Hospitalization: A Randomized Trial', *Medical Care*, **37**, pp. 5–14.

Towle, A. (1998), 'Continuing Medical Education: Changes in Health Care and Continuing Medical Education for the 21st Century', *British Medical Journal*, **316**, 24 January, pp. 301–304.

CHAPTER 14

Patient Compliance: A Complex Picture Emerges

Dr Faiz Kermani

As will have become apparent from the numerous contributions to this book, patient compliance can be examined from many different angles – technical, social and economic to cite just a few. In their own ways the authors have attempted to highlight the range of factors that influence how patients comply with their medicines in order to illustrate the complexity of the subject.

One of the initial difficulties of working in this field is that there exist a multitude of definitions and phrases that relate to the phenomenon of compliance. As communication plays an important role in improving the compliance of patients with their medicines, all interested parties must have confidence in the basic terminology being used. This is critical if different approaches to addressing compliance issues are to be compared, particularly in an international context where translations may be required – Chapter 2 provides a 'View from the Real World'.

In reality, the range of factors that influence patient compliance should not be surprising, as there are occasions when we find ourselves as the 'patient'. As one chapter author rightly points out, can we honestly say that we have always complied fully with every tablet of every prescription and have always finished the course of treatment? The truth is that everyone is non-compliant to some degree. Indeed, there are even cases of 'overcompliance', where a patient consumes more drugs than prescribed in the belief that more will be better.

Perhaps if we look at our own experiences as 'the patient' we may gain more of an understanding as to how people are influenced when they take their medicines. As described in Chapter 5, a French study has highlighted how education levels can affect patients' attitudes to the advice received from their physicians. Furthermore, due to the availability of the Internet it is all too easy to come across information that appears to conflict with the advice of the doctor or pharmacist. What is needed is a less theoretical and more practical approach to the subject – in essence, we must focus on 'real-world non-compliance'.

The nature of a medicine and its effects can have a strong bearing on the degree of patient compliance. Patients expect a drug to treat a disease or symptoms, not to provide discomfort or further symptoms. It has been observed that these opinions can be affected to a surprising extent by the patient's lifestyle, education level, socioeconomic status and general beliefs.

Apart from the way in which patients may think about the medicines, the formulation (for example, capsules) and presentation (for example, push-through blister pack) prescribed should suit the patients in terms of their lifestyle or age or health condition. For example, the elderly may be physically unable to open certain types of presentations such as bottles containing drops, where they must unscrew the top. Children may also have difficulties taking certain types of product or may not wish to have them administered because of a general dislike of the particular presentation.

It is the harsh realities of modern healthcare, where budgets limit the care available to patients, which have also driven an interest in patient compliance. In countries where the government burden is high for funding public healthcare, there is a strong incentive for them to try to reduce the per capita cost. Patient non-compliance is now being closely examined within an economic framework as healthcare providers assess how improvements will enable them to better allocate their limited resources. However, as has been shown in Chapter 3, extreme care must be taken when using economic tools in the field of compliance. The limitations in methodology can complicate the interpretation of studies and it is important to note that medical expenditures do not always increase because of poor compliance.

Patient compliance is increasingly recognized as a problem extending beyond following physicians' instructions and, therefore, solutions require cooperation between all those involved in healthcare delivery and usage. In fact, the World Health Organization has called for a multidisciplinary approach towards improving patient compliance that involves health professionals, researchers, health planners and policy-makers. In particular, the manufacturers of medicines can do more to improve the situation. These companies have the resources and commercial interest to proactively support the patient compliance effort by partnering with physicians and healthcare teams. Despite the technology being used to enhance patient compliance, physician–patient relationships remain the key driver of good patient compliance.

It is also important to appreciate the role of the pharmacist, particularly in countries where they continue to be involved in the actual preparation of the final product that patients receive. As described in Chapter 7, in Japan it is common for dispensing pharmacists to grind tablets into powders to assist patients who have difficulties when swallowing tablets. Thus pharmaceutical companies are expected to provide them with information on the stability of tablets after the grinding process, even though the companies may not have originally intended their products to be ground up.

Nevertheless, there is an important role for a technological approach in improving the situation. A number of exciting and innovative technologies are being applied to the delivery of drug products, but, as has been noted, the form that a particular medicine takes can have a major bearing on the attitude of the patient to the treatment. Pharmaceutical scientists and others involved in product development are exploring a range of technologies to determine how they can make pharmaceuticals more patient-friendly and gain a patient's confidence in using a medicine.

Due to their convenience, most patients prefer oral dosage forms, yet the nature of the molecules currently in development often renders them inappropriate for development as oral dosage forms. This has often restricted products to injectable forms, which are unpopular with patients. If drugs can be delivered non-invasively, they can greatly improve patient compliance and this has led to the development of such approaches as dermal patches, inhalation devices and nasal sprays. There are also advances being made within the field of injections, and the goal of developing painless needles is becoming more realistic.

There is a growing role for interactive communication technologies in compliance programmes, and a number of published studies have demonstrated the value of these approaches. Technologies such as Interactive Voice Response (IVR), interactive text messaging (Short Message Service or SMS text) and the Internet and e-mail can be used to provide reminder messages and to deliver education and counselling to increase patients' involvement with their treatment (see Chapter 10).

When examining the issues concerning patient compliance we must be aware that up until now we have restricted our discussions to established mainstream Western medicine. However, the reality is that a growing number of patients are using complementary medicines and so their use must be factored into discussions concerning compliance. Although this is a feature of many Western markets, it is also important for emerging countries, which are growing in importance as healthcare markets. Unfortunately we were unable to address compliance issues regarding complementary medicines in depth for this edition of the book but we hope that they can be covered in the future.

For example, in the rapidly evolving Chinese market, traditional medicines make up between 30–50 per cent of total medicinal consumption (WHO, 2003). Self-medication is popular, and a recent survey found that usage of either traditional or Western medicines varied considerably depending on the condition being treated (Zhang and Zhou, 2005). What was interesting was the satisfaction ratings of those surveyed. In all conditions studied, the consumers rated traditional medicines highly, even for conditions where Western medication had higher usage levels in the country (ibid.). Such findings illustrate how patient compliance cannot be ignored wherever healthcare is examined in the world.

We must appreciate that there is no universally applicable means of improving compliance. What works in one particular therapeutic area may be inappropriate for another and what works in one country or region may be of little use elsewhere. What we can conclude is that, by having an open and proactive approach to compliance issues, we may be able to draw upon a range of options from different scenarios and modify them to suit the particular situation that faces us. It is hoped that this book will serve to stimulate discussion of the issues surrounding patient compliance and that, as the field grows, new approaches can be covered in future editions.

REFERENCES

WHO (2003), 'Traditional Medicine', *World Health Organization Fact Sheet No. 134*, at: http://www.who.int/mediacentre/factsheets/fs134/en.

Zhang, Y. and Zhou, M. (2005), 'Unfolding China's Consumer Potential', *World Pharmaceutical Frontiers*, 1, pp. 20–23, available at: http://www.worldpharmaceuticals.net.

Index